Advances in Medical Education and Training

Edited by Zouhair O. Amarin

Published in London, United Kingdom

Advances in Medical Education and Training
http://dx.doi.org/10.5772/intechopen.114626
Edited by Zouhair O. Amarin

Contributors
Ayikoru Jackline, Aysel Baser, Cristina Miyazaki, Ebtihaj T. Nafea, Eduardo Miyazaki, Felix Bongomin, Giovanna Miyazaki, Hatice Şahin, Henry Tulgan, Maxwell Opwonya, Mehdi Afkar, Parisa Shojaei, Pebalo Francis Pebolo, Raymond Otim, Seyed Mansour Razavi, Vida Seifouri, Ömer Faruk Sönmez

First published in London, United Kingdom, 2024 by IntechOpen
IntechOpen is the global imprint of INTECHOPEN LIMITED, registered in England and Wales, registration number: 11086078, 167-169 Great Portland Street, London, W1W 5PF, United Kingdom

British Library Cataloguing-in-Publication Data
A catalogue record for this book is available from the British Library

Additional hard and PDF copies can be obtained from orders@intechopen.com

Advances in Medical Education and Training
Edited by Zouhair O. Amarin
p. cm.

This title is part of the Education and Human Development Book Series, Volume 18
Topic: Education
Series Editor: Katherine Meltzoff
Topic Editor: Delfín Ortega-Sánchez and Carlos Pérez-González

Print ISBN 978-0-85014-108-5
Online ISBN 978-0-85014-109-2
eBook (PDF) ISBN 978-0-85014-110-8
ISSN 2755-9513

For EU product safety concerns :
IN TECH d.o.o., Prolaz Marije Krucifikse Kozulić 3, 51000 Rijeka, Croatia,
info@intechopen.com or visit our website at intechopen.com.

IntechOpen Book Series

Education and Human Development

Volume 18

Aims and Scope of the Series

Education and Human Development is an interdisciplinary research area that aims to shed light on topics related to both learning and development. This Series is intended for researchers, practitioners, and students who are interested in understanding more about these fields and their applications.

Meet the Series Editor

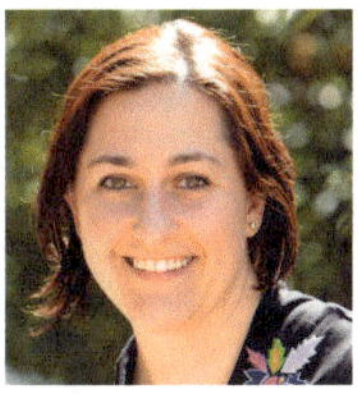

Katherine Meltzoff received her BA in Psychology from Trinity College, in Connecticut, USA and her Ph.D. in Experimental Psychology from the University of California, San Diego. She completed her postdoctoral work at the Yale Child Study Center with Dr. James McPartland. Dr. Meltzoff' doctoral dissertation explored neural correlates of reward anticipation to social versus nonsocial stimuli in children with and without autism spectrum disorders (ASD). She has been a faculty member at the University of California, Riverside in the School of Education since 2016. Her research focuses on translational studies to explore the reward system in ASD, as well as how anxiety contributes to social challenges in ASD. She also investigates how behavioral interventions affect neural activity, behavior, and school performance in children with ASD. She is also involved in the diagnosis of children with ASD and is a licensed clinical psychologist in California. She is the Assistant Director of the SEARCH Center at UCR and is a faculty member in the Graduate Program in Neuroscience.

Meet the Volume Editor

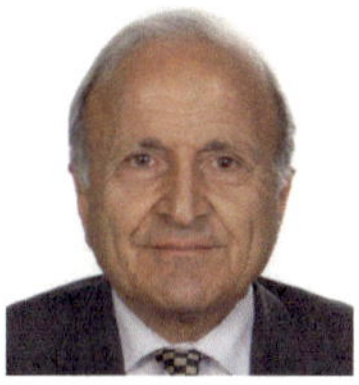

Renowned obstetrician and gynecologist Professor Zouhair Amarin was previously employed at the Jordan University of Science and Technology and is currently at the University of Jordan. He has been a lecturer at the University of Glasgow, Scotland, a senior lecturer at the University of Nottingham, England, and the dean of the Faculty of Medicine, Mutah University, Jordan. He is a fellow of the Faculty of Public Health, London, and the Royal College of Obstetricians and Gynaecologists. He also has master's degrees in medical education from Maastricht, Netherlands, and medical science from Glasgow, Scotland. Developing microsurgical epididymis sperm aspiration and discovering a surgical treatment for critical ovarian hyperstimulation syndrome, Professor Amarin is a pioneer in the field of in vitro fertilization. He has published more than 130 papers, edited numerous books, written several book chapters, and received eight awards.

Contents

Preface **XIII**

Section 1
Continued Professional Development **1**

Chapter 1 **3**
The Evolution of Continuing Medical Education in the United States
by Henry Tulgan

Chapter 2 **13**
Physicians' Mental Health: Is It Possible to Tackle the Problem throughout Academic Education?
by Eduardo Miyazaki, Giovanna Miyazaki and M. Cristina Miyazaki

Section 2
Professionalism in Medical Education **25**

Chapter 3 **27**
Professional Behavior in Medical Practice
by Vida Seifouri

Chapter 4 **55**
Professional Values and Ethics in Medical Education
by Ebtihaj T. Nafea

Section 3
Contemporary Teaching Methods **67**

Chapter 5 **69**
Immersive Explorations: Transformative Experiences in Inter-Professional Education through Scenario-Based Learning
by Aysel Başer, Ömer Faruk Sönmez and Hatice Şahin

Chapter 6 **91**
Triple Taxon Test/Technique: An Innovative Method for Self-Learning and Self-Evaluation in Health Problems
by Seyed Mansour Razavi, Mehdi Afkar and Parisa Shojaei

Chapter 7 **105**
Medical Education Technology in Resource-Limited Settings
by Pebalo Francis Pebolo, Ayikoru Jackline, Maxwell Opwonya, Raymond Otim and Felix Bongomin

Preface

The ever-changing landscape of medical education demands a persistent commitment to quality, flexibility, and creativity. This volume compiles a wide range of viewpoints and research findings, providing insight into important topics that are now changing medical education.

In Chapter 1, "The Evolution of Continuing Medical Education in the United States", Professor Henry Tulgan offers a thorough examination of the advances in Continuing Medical Education (CME) during the previous few decades. This chapter examines the development of continuous education and shows how it has adapted to the changing needs of healthcare providers and patients.

Chapter 2, "Physicians' Mental Health: Is It Possible to Tackle the Problem throughout Academic Education?" by Assistant Professor Eduardo Miyazaki et al., addresses the important topic of medical practitioners' mental health. It discusses the stresses that come with being a doctor along with methods for including mental health support in the medical education curriculum.

Chapter 3, "Professional Behavior in Medical Practice" by Dr. Vida Seifouri, examines the fundamental elements of professional behavior and emphasizes the value of honesty, compassion, and open communication in fostering a culture of trust and efficiency in the medical field.

Chapter 4, "Professional Values and Ethics in Medical Education" by Assistant Professor Ebtihaj T. Nafea, examines the critical role that ethics and values play in forming medical professionals. This chapter provides a framework for moral decision-making in medical education and discusses the ethical issues that medical practitioners and students must deal with.

In Chapter 5, "Immersive Explorations: Transformative Experiences in Inter-Professional Education through Scenario-Based Learning", Assistant Professor Aysel Başer et al. discuss the consequences of teaching techniques, highlighting the advantages of scenario-based learning for fostering critical thinking and teamwork among medical professionals from different specialties.

Chapter 6, "Triple Taxon Test/Technique: An Innovative Method for Self-Learning and Self-Evaluation in Health Problems" by Assistant Professor Parisa Shojaei et al., presents a novel strategy for self-directed learning and evaluation. The Triple Taxon Test is introduced in this chapter as a tool to help medical students better evaluate themselves and take charge of their education.

In Chapter 7, "Medical Education Technology in Resource-Limited Settings", Dr. Pebalo Francis Pebolo et al address the particular difficulties encountered in settings with limited resources. This chapter focuses on innovative approaches and technology advancements that are improving the effectiveness and accessibility of medical education in underdeveloped areas.

I would like to thank all the authors for their invaluable efforts and contributions, and to express my sincere gratitude to Ms. Romina Rovan Bakarcic at IntechOpen for all her help, support, and advice.

It is our hope that this compilation of chapters will prove to be an invaluable aid for instructors, learners, and professionals, providing motivation and useful direction for managing the intricacies of medical education.

Zouhair O. Amarin
Professor,
Department of Obstetrics and Gynaecology,
University of Jordan,
Amman, Jordan

Section 1

Continued Professional Development

Chapter 1

The Evolution of Continuing Medical Education in the United States

Henry Tulgan

Abstract

For centuries, medical education was obtained by serving an apprenticeship with established physicians or obtaining a degree from an established University. Incorporating new knowledge and skills into one's practice requires a commitment to lifetime learning. Traditional Continuing Medical Education (CME) had no formal requirements for many centuries, although there is ample documentation of efforts to make certain that lifetime learning was being followed, dating back to at least the fourteenth century. Although CME was recognized as one of the silos of medical education for many years, the current system for accreditation of CME in the United States only dates back to 1968. The establishment of and current operation of this system will be presented in this manuscript.

Keywords: Continuing Medical Education, lifelong learning, historical development, present status in the United States, Interprofessional Continuing Education

1. Introduction

Continuing Medical Education (CME) has a long, uneven history. For centuries, physicians began their careers in medicine by serving as apprentices to established practitioners or by obtaining a degree from an established university. After starting practice and meeting new and more complex problems, physicians soon realized that graduation from a formal process of training marked not just the beginning of healthcare delivery but the need for another phase of the educational process: the need to incorporate new skills and knowledge into their lives continually and thus to make a commitment to CME [1].

Records dating back to the fourteenth century show that the City of Venice, Italy, required physicians and surgeons to maintain their competence by attending lectures, doing dissections, and presenting case studies, a mandate that lasted until 1802. Practitioners were required to swear an oath before the judicial authority that outlined the standards of practice to be followed and to promise to refrain from certain unethical or unseemly practices [2]. Whether or not these laws were followed is unclear, but they existed for five centuries. Other CME opportunities did exist from the sixteenth to the eighteenth centuries in European cities that contained medical schools where physicians had opportunities to attend lectures and dissections in order to improve their knowledge and skills [1]. Such opportunities did not exist for many practitioners in more rural areas of Europe and colonial America, where the first medical school did not open until 1782 in Massachusetts after the Revolutionary War. Sporadic CME presentations that followed are documented but were few and far between [3–5].

2. CME in the United States

Despite the subsequent growth of medical schools in the United States, they and national medical organizations were slow to mobilize to address the need for CME. Throughout the late eighteenth and nineteenth centuries, CME was offered predominantly by local county and state medical societies. At the beginning of the twentieth century, Sir William Osler and the 1907 McCormack report to the American Medical Association (AMA) independently emphasized the necessity for more attention to CME [6].

However, neither of these had much immediate impact on medical schools and national organizations, although several demonstration projects were briefly undertaken. Even in the early twentieth century, when advances were being made in undergraduate and graduate medical education, CME lagged behind and for the most part, continued to be the province of local, county, and state societies [7–13].

To address the challenges of educating physicians far from urban areas or near the 81 medical schools in the United States, a significant innovation in CME began in the early part of the second half of the twentieth century. A pilot program was initiated at the Albany NY Medical College in 1955 via its powerful FM radio station atop Mt. Greylock, the highest mountain in nearby Massachusetts, using amateur radio operators. It reached participating hospitals in New York, New Jersey, Massachusetts, Vermont, and Connecticut. Faculty were recruited from 23 medical schools across the United States and Canada [14–17].

Although the Albany program ceased operating in 1981, it was followed by a host of interactive teaching modalities that have expanded even more since the COVID-19 pandemic.

Organized medicine finally began to accredit CME in a more formal manner in 1968. The AMA's Council on Medical Education first assumed this role and then was succeeded by a Liaison Committee for Continuing Medical Education (LCCME) in 1976. LCCME was not successful in its operations because other organizations involved in medical education felt that they should have significant roles to play in CME accreditation and were not represented.

AMA transiently resumed its supervisory by forming a standing Advisory Committee on Continuing Medical Education and, in 1968, developed the AMA Physician's Recognition Award and Credit System. It defined CME as nonpromotional learning activities certified for credit prior to the activity by an organization authorized by the credit system owner or nonpromotional learning activities for which the credit system owner directly awards credit. It also defined activities that are ineligible for AMA PRA credit. These include:

Clinical experience
Charity or mission work
Mentoring
Surveying

Serving on a committee, council, task force, board, house of delegates, or other professional workgroup
Passing examinations that are not integrated with a certified activity.

It developed categories of AMA PRA Credit, Eligibility for Credit, AMA monitoring, and withdrawal of privilege to designate credit. It developed core requirements for certifying activities and format—specific ones: these are:

Live activities
Enduring materials
Journal-based CME
Test-item writing
Manuscript review
Performance improvement CME
Internet point of care learning
Other.

And listed activities that could receive credit directly:

Teaching at a live activity
Publishing articles
Poster presentations
Medically related advanced degree
American Board of Medical Specialists (ABMS) member board certification and Maintenance of Certification (MOC)
ACGME accredited education
AMA international conference recognition
AMA PRA credit system international agreements.

Finally, in 1981, medical educators cooperatively formed the Accreditation Council for Continuing Medical Education. Those seven member organizations are:

The American Board of Medical Specialists (ABMS)
The American Hospital Association (AHA)
The American Medical Association (AMA)
The Association of American Medical Colleges (AAMC)
The Association for Hospital Medical Education (AHME)
The Council of Medical Specialty Societies (CMSS, now CMS)
The Federation of State Medical Boards (FSMB) [18].

Whereas its predecessors were unsuccessful in accomplishing a role that was acceptable to all involved in the credit process for CME, ACCME has done so for over 40 years. Jointly with the AMA, ACCME promulgated its definition of CME.

"Continuing Medical Education (CME) consists of educational activities that serve to maintain, develop or increase the knowledge, skills and professional performance and relationships that a physician uses to provide services for patients, the public or the profession. The content of CME is that body of knowledge and skills generally recognized and accepted by the profession as within the basic medical sciences, the discipline of clinical medicine, and the provision of health care to the public."

This definition is widely accepted by the profession.

In 2022, the most recent Data Report by ACCME reported 1620 accredited providers who offered approximately 230,000 accredited educational activities. Although over the past few years, the number of providers has fallen because of hospital closures, provider mergers, and economic issues, the number of AMA Category 1 Credits offered, Physician Interactions, and Other Learner Interactions continue to increase.

Although the Albany Medical College Program had been discontinued, it had been succeeded by numerous telelectures, one-way and two-way television programs, and the like. The pandemic introduced numerous presentations available to learners, primarily via ZOOM. Such media has increased attendee numbers and remains widely used despite the end of pandemic restrictions.

There are multitudes of reasons for this success. Among them is the growth of Hospitalists, which causes many physicians to have less presence in hospital settings and the convenience of attending learning opportunities from their offices or even off-hours from their homes. Remote faculty become available from many sources. A further innovation has been the development of a "hybrid" format where some learners attend in person and others remotely. Detractors of remote learning decry the lack of opportunity for in-person attendees to chat or discuss presentations with peers and faculty.

The US CME enterprise is financially very successful: In 2022, the Grand total income was $3387, 101, 116, reflecting Registration Fees, Commercial Support, Advertising and exhibit income, Government grants, and Private donations [18].

3. The survey process

Organizations that provide either state or national CME accreditation undergo a three-part process: they submit a Self-Study document along with a number of their activities labeled "Performance-in Practice" (also known as Activity files) for review by a team of two Surveyors. The Surveyors then interview the Provider, increasingly by ZOOM, thereby obviating a need for travel.

The specific areas covered in the updated Self Study are:

Mission
Program analysis
Program improvements
Educational needs
Designed to change
Appropriate formats
Competencies
Analyzes change

and a number of standards and policies

Standard 1: ensure content is valid
Standard 2: prevent commercial bias and marketing in accredited continuing education
Standard 3: identify, mitigate, and disclose relevant financial relationships
Standard 4: manage commercial support appropriately
Standard 5: manage ancillary activities

Accreditation statement policy
CME activity and attendance records retention policy

Performance-in practice submissions reflect the nature of the organization being surveyed.

Accreditation is granted to multiple learning formats derived from the AMA PRA. These include:

Enduring material
Live courses
Regularly scheduled series
Journal CME/CE
Other/blended learning
Performance/quality improvement
Committee learning
Manuscript review
Test-item writing
Internet searching and learning
Learning from teaching.

The findings of the Survey Team are reviewed in a tripartite process first by a member of the ACCME Accreditation Review Committee and presented to the Committee for a vote. It is further reviewed by the Accreditation Decision Committee of the Board of Directors, and the decision is conveyed to the organization.

Organizations that are newly applying for accreditation, if successful, receive a two-year level of accreditation entitled Provisional, after which they are again surveyed. Two levels of accreditation then may be achieved: a Four-Year status, which may also require Progress Notes if any of the replies are unsatisfactory, which are further reviewed, or a Six-Year level of Accreditation with Commendation that is granted after an applicant answers additional Criteria from a menu that encompasses:

Promotes team-based education
Engages teams
Engages patients/public
Engages students

Addresses public health priorities
Advances data use
Addresses population health
Collaborates effectively

Enhances skills
Optimizes communication skills
Optimizes technical/procedural skills
Creates individual learning plans
Utilizes support strategies

Demonstrates educational leadership
Engages in research/scholarship
Supports CPD for CME team-based demonstrates creativity/innovation

Achieves outcomes
Improves performance-in improves healthcare quality
Improves patient/community health

It is required to demonstrate compliance with any seven criteria of the organization's choice plus one criterion from achieves outcomes. No leeway is allowed in the responses for providers seeking commendation in the form of progress notes. The vast majority of providers achieve a four-year accreditation, with less than 10% acquiring commendation.

It must be noted that in addition to the 155 medical schools in the United States and 17 in Canada that award the MD degree, there are an additional 41 accredited medical colleges that grant the degree of Doctor of Osteopathic Medicine (DO) that are accredited by the American Osteopathic Association's (AOA) Commission on Osteopathic College Accreditation [19]. Approximately 19% of practicing physicians in the US hold that degree. There has been increasing integration of both undergraduate [20] and graduate medical education between allopathic and osteopathic training, and many osteopaths, following their graduate training, become certified by ABMS and obtain CME largely through ACCME. As of this moment, despite that there have been some attempts to do so [21], there has not yet been a successful merger in the CME functions of the AOA and AMA, and so the AOA has a parallel accreditation process to ACCME's. An increasing number of osteopathic medical colleges have applied for ACCME certification and may award CME to allopathic attendees.

4. The role of academic medicine

Academic medicine began to play a significant role in CME with the establishment of the Society of Medical College Directors of Continuing Medical Education in 1976. It developed a publication, Mobius, in 1981, which was retitled The Journal of Continuing Education in the Health Professions in 1988 and renamed itself the Society for Academic Continuing Medical Education in 1998. Although the organization emphasized educational advances, by 1995, it received a request from the Association of American Medical Colleges (AAMC) for a statement on CME and entered into working groups with ACCME, and participated in its restructuring process in 1996; SACME now recognized for its commitment to being the leading academic society that advances the field of continuing education and professional development in the health professions in the best interests of clinicians, patients, and communities. SACME now describes its mission as:

Health equity
Practice and value of CPD/CE
Clinician practice and wellbeing
Patient care and health of the public.

SACME reaches its members in the academic medical community via its additional publications CE News and Intercom. Utilizing a grant from ACCME, SACME has developed the CE Educator's Toolkit, an accessible resource for educators containing best practices and guidelines to deliver effective continuing education [22].

5. Discussion

ACCME is defined as accredited providers and organizations that offer CME to primarily national or international audiences.

In addition to its directly accredited providers in the United States, many of which are Medical Colleges, Academic Medical Centers, State Medical Societies, large member Specialty Societies, and corporate entities in or associated with the field of healthcare.

ACCME collaborates with 32 state and territorial medical societies, "state accredited providers," several of which accredit CME in contiguous ones. As an example, the Commonwealth of Massachusetts also accredits neighboring Connecticut and Rhode Island. The nomenclature for such providers is accreditation by ACCME Recognized Accreditors. Some entities within those states may receive that level of accreditation instead of national accreditation.

This is accomplished by a concept of Substantial Equivalency propagated early this century that such accreditation is based on shared principles and values. State Societies review processes are similar to those outlined for national accreditation.

The results of the State Societies processes are then entered into ACCME's Program and Activities Reporting System (PARS) for the convenience of the learners and licensing boards.

The third group of Providers are Jointly accredited ones that focus on continuing education by and for healthcare teams. These providers are accredited by Joint Accreditation for Interprofessional Continuing Education.

ACCME works in concert with the AMA to simplify and align its expectations for accredited CME activities that it certifies for AMA Category 1 Credit.

ACCME also cooperates with ABMS member boards to simplify the process of Maintenance of Certification (MOC), which is another convenience for its learner audience.

The US Food and Drug Administration collaborates with ACCME via its Opioid Quality Payment Risk Evaluation and Mitigation Strategy.

CMS, formerly CMSS (The Centers for Medicare and Medicaid Services) Quality Payment Program includes, as an improvement activity, accredited CME.

The development of Joint Accreditation for Interprofessional Continuing Education allows for the accreditation of activities specifically designed to promote collaborative interprofessional activities in healthcare delivery.

Collaborative programs with international accreditors who have shared principles allow for continuing professional development for clinicians and teams worldwide.

ACCME has increasingly taken a leadership role with CME representatives from many countries. It played a significant role in creating the International Academy for CPD Accreditation in 2013, whose goal is to facilitate peer-to-peer support for leaders of CPD/CME accreditation systems while encouraging networking, mentoring, and interactions about common issues.

Through its principle of Substantial Equivalency, six organizations outside the United States are recognized by ACCME as equals:

The Royal College of Physicians and Surgeons of Canada
The Canadian Committee on Accreditation of Continuing Medical Education
European Board for Accreditation of CE for Health Professionals

The Oman Medical Specialty Board as part of the Ministry of Health of the Sultanate
The Qatar Council for Health Practitioners
The Federation of the German Chambers of Physicians.

ACCME also directly accredits organizations outside the United States that undergo its Survey Process. These include organizations in the United Kingdom, Canada, Korea, Pakistan, Qatar, Saudi Arabia, and Chile.

6. Conclusion

In its 42 years of existence, ACCME has accomplished elevating CME to reach a level of expertise in the United States that is on a level offered in both undergraduate and graduate medical education that had not previously existed.

In the United States, CME has survived and rebounded from the negative effects of the pandemic and has developed new and exciting modes of delivery.

In addition, ACCME has taken a leadership role in international CME, which has also profited from its expertise.

CME in the United States and increasingly worldwide is thriving despite the fact that changes lagged behind those at the levels of undergraduate and graduate medical education. Its advances over the past 42 years have progressed so that CME has become equal with medical school and graduate education programs.

Changes that are continually present in healthcare will continue to present challenges in review of activities for scientific integrity. Issues surrounding commercial support will continue to challenge Surveyors and Reviewers and the emerging role of Artificial Intelligence will present new ones.

The strengthened CME community looks forward to meeting these challenges in the United States and worldwide.

Author details

Henry Tulgan
University of Massachusetts Chan Medical School, Worcester, MA, USA

*Address all correspondence to: htulgan@gmail.com

References

[1] Lyons AS, Petrucelli R. Medicine and Illustrated History. New York: Abdrdale Press; 1987

[2] Ell SR. Five hundred years of specialty certification and compulsory continuing medical education. Venice 13300-1801. Journal of the American Medical Association. 1984;**251**:752-753

[3] Bergin P. A History of Worcester District Medical Society. Worcester, MA: Deerfield Press; 1994

[4] Burrage WI. A History of the Massachusetts Medical Society, 1781-1922. Privately Printed. p. 1923

[5] Smith AM. Historical Address > Berkshire Medical Society Centennial Dinner. Historical Archives, Berkshire District Medical Society; 1887 [Accessed 2004]

[6] McGovern JP, Roland CG. William Osler: The Continuing Education. Springfield, IL: Thomas; 1969

[7] Aghababian R, Tulgan H. The evolution of continuing medical education: The Massachusetts experience. Berkshire Medical Journal. 2004;**12**:3-7

[8] Maryland Medical Society. Documentary history of philanthropy: "MedChi." Available from: http://www.medchi.org [Accessed: December 12, 2023]

[9] Bruce JB. Postgraduate education in Michigan. Journal of the Michigan State Medical Society. 1937;**36**:172

[10] Clark JC. The Development of Physician Continuation Education. Iowa City: University of Iowa Press; 1966

[11] Wentz DK. Continuing Medical Education: Looking Back, Planning Ahead. Hanover, NH: Dartmouth Press; 2011

[12] Medical Society of the County of Kings. Brooklyn Medical Journal. Reprint. London, England: Forgotten Books; 2013

[13] Shepherd GR. History of continuation medical education in the United States since 1930. Journal of Medical Education. 1960;**35**:748

[14] Woolsey FM. Two years of experience with two-way radio conferences for postgraduate medical education. Journal of Medical Education. 1958;**33**(6):474-482

[15] Woolsey FM. Two-way radio conferences for postgraduate medical education. Four years of experience with a new method of presentation. Canadian Medical Association Journal. 1960;**82**:717-719

[16] Woolsey FM. Two-way radio and its advantages. Annals of the New York Academy of Sciences. 1967;**142**(2):424-427

[17] Tulgan H. The Albany two-way radio conferences, 1955-1981: A retrospective look at a program providing interactive continuing medical education at a distance. Journal of Continuing Education in the Health Professions. 2014;**34**(3):196-198

[18] Accreditation Council for Continuing Medical Education (ACCME). Available from: https://www.accme.org/ [Accessed: December 1, 2023]

[19] American Osteopathic Association (AOA). Available from: https://osteopathic.org/ [Accessed: December 13, 2023]

[20] Tulgan H, DeMarco W, Pugnaire MP, Buser B. Joint clinical clerkships for osteopathic and allopathic medical students: New England's experience. JAOA. 2004;**104**(5):212-214

[21] Plungas GS, Tulgan H, DeMarco WJ, Aghababian RV. Accomplishing dual credit for a conference. Journal of Continuing Education in the Health Professions. 2001;**21**(3):182-186

[22] The Society for Academic Continuing Medical Education (SACME). Available from: https://sacme.org/ [Accessed: December 14, 2023]

Chapter 2

Physicians' Mental Health: Is It Possible to Tackle the Problem throughout Academic Education?

Eduardo Miyazaki, Giovanna Miyazaki and M. Cristina Miyazaki

Abstract

Changes over the years require adaptation to thrive in today's academic and professional scenarios. Teachers of future healthcare professionals face new challenges daily, like artificial intelligence and its impact on learning, helping young students to keep focused, using the best available data and good teaching/ learning resources, making evidence-based decisions. As new demands arise, some of the old ones are still present, challenging students, teachers, and professionals. When it comes to medical education, learning how to deal with professional's mental health is still an issue. This chapter aims to discuss strategies to improve physicians and medical students 'abilities to cope with stress and mental health issues, and its impacts on their life and on the lives of their patients and families.

Keywords: mental health, medical students, physicians mental health, stress, healthcare professionals

1. Introduction

Science and technology develop fast, and it is possible to encounter something new almost every day. Perhaps one of the latest technological developments is the application of Artificial Intelligence to healthcare services [1]. Keeping up to date is no easy task, and time and energy consuming but fortunately as soon as something new is launched there are studies in the area applying and assessing its use and its impact [2]. A high-pressure working environment, long hours on the job, limited resources, restricted autonomy, and several other obstacles and dilemmas, may turn physicians more vulnerable to high levels of stress, burnout, and mental disorders [3–5].

Being a physician is considered a rewarded and sought-after profession. But there are stressors associated with medical education and the practice of medicine that raises concerns about medical students and physicians' mental health. And those concerns increased after COVID-19 [5–9].

High levels of stress, burnout, suicidal ideation, and suicide have been frequently reported among medical students and physicians, leading organizations from different countries to issue "calls to action, demanding a greater focus on physician mental health within training programs, workplaces, and health service more broadly". Beyond the concern about professionals' mental health, several studies have shown its negative impact on patient care (e.g. medical incidents) [5].

Any mental disorder may affect medical students and physicians, but depression and anxiety are the most prevalent. A German study among first year medical students [10] identified a prevalence of 4.7% of major depression, 5.8% of depressive symptoms, 4.4% of anxiety symptoms, 1.9% of panic disorder, and 15.7% of psychosomatic complaints. Although these results were higher than those of the general population, medical students fared better when compared to those on advanced medical training (e.g. residency. The same study also identified that 10.7% of the first-year medical students used psychotropic substances regularly, 5.1% used medication for anxiety, 4.6 to improve sleep, 4.4% for depression and 3.1% to improve cognitive performance.

A systematic review and meta-analysis estimated a prevalence of 28.8% of depression or depressive symptoms among residents [4]. A study with Dutch physicians showed a prevalence of 42% of work-related fatigue, 29% of depression, 24% of anxiety, 15% of PTSD (Post-Traumatic Stress Disorder), 15% of stress complaints and 6% of burnout [11]. Those numbers are situated above the prevalence observed in the general population [12].

Anderson et al. [13] analyzed data from Dutch medical school applications to assess the association between becoming a physician and the use of prescription drugs and receiving mental health treatment. The authors concluded that "becoming a physician increases the use of antidepressants, anxiolytics, opioids, and sedatives" and that the use is larger among female physicians.

Since the prevalence of stress, burnout and mental disorders is high among medical students, residents, and physicians', data from several studies and organization emphasize the need for prevention at the beginning and during medical school [3]. This shows that something must be done to tackle the problem [14].

Even though the burden of mental illness in medical students and professionals has been an issue for a long time, not enough has been done to improve the situation. This raises a few questions about the topic. Is this a problem inherent to the profession? Is it related to the work context, like long hours, high pressure on the job, life and death decision making, high responsibilities and little room for error? Is it possible to help medical students and physicians to better cope with the problems associated with the practice of medicine?

Mental health problems are not inherent to studying and practicing medicine but related to other variables as well. Studies about burnout among health care professionals show that many other variables have a significant role when it comes to this, and workplace is an example. Physicians working in hospitals (inpatient settings) are more vulnerable to mental health problems than their colleagues working in outpatient settings [15]. Also, when it comes to COVID-19, frontline workers showed higher prevalence of burnout when compared to second line workers [16]. Besides workplace, other variables were associated with high levels of burnout, like administrative tasks, harassment at work, sacrifice of personal time and regretting decisions regarding patients [17].

It is safe to say that seeking mental health is an issue when it comes to healthcare professionals. Braquehais and Vargas-Cáceres [18] pointed several reasons that preclude those professional from seeking mental health care. The most frequent ones are related to an increased sense of invulnerability, perfectionism, a proneness to trying to cope alone, insecurity and stigma related to mental distress and fear of licensure problems when facing a mental health condition. Although there are some difficulties, not seeking help could pose a higher threat to both professionals and patients.

Treating mental health problems is possible and should be done, but there is also need for prevention. Preventing these problems and teaching students and physicians how to deal with them could be a better solution on the long run. A recent study among Portuguese medical students found that adaptive coping, academic engagement, and social support were inversely correlated with the intention of dropping out of medical school. The study also concluded that burnout was associated with lack of social support, depression, anxiety, stress, and non-functional coping strategies [19]. This is very promising since it shows a few variables to look for and to try to develop throughout medical school.

When it comes to medical education there are a few struggles that need to be addressed. A qualitative exploratory study [20] highlighted emotions, academic and family related problems as the main themes that undergraduates were struggling with. Emotional problems, for example, were related to conflict with friends. Time management was associated with academic problems when living with the family (e.g. distractions, such as guests). Interesting enough, this study shows that, unlike previous ones, the increased workload and highly demanding nature of medical education were causing less stress among students than family related problems. This suggests that social skills development, emotional regulation and adapting to certain contexts may be more important than previously thought and highlights the importance of developing these skills to solve such problems.

2. How to improve medical students and physicians 'mental health?

To help students cope with many problems faced throughout medical school and to prevent future mental health issues among physicians, there are a few programs that deserve attention.

2.1 Mentoring

Mentorship or mentoring programs in medical education date from the early 1990s. Their aim is to provide medical students with research opportunities, advice on career decisions, and to facilitate personal and professional development [21].

Mentoring aims to support, guide, and help students through a relationship with a mentor. A mentor is usually someone with more experience (e.g. a professor) that may help and guide the mentee (medical student) through different situations, such as: career development, interpersonal difficulties, personal and professional growth, and other issues [22, 23].

Although the term mentoring may be used in different contexts and with different meanings, its role during medical education may be better understood by Johnson's definition [24]: "Mentoring is a personal and reciprocal relationship in which a more experienced (usually older) faculty member acts as a guide, role model, teacher, sponsor of a less experienced (usually younger) student or faculty member. A mentor provides the mentee with knowledge, advice, counsel, challenge, and support in the mentee's pursuit of becoming a full member of a particular profession" (p. 23).

Using a qualitative approach, the strengths, and fragilities of a group mentoring program from a Brazilian medical school were assessed with mentors and mentees [23]. The strengths included: creating bonds between group members, the possibility to express feelings in a safe and welcoming environment, benefits for mentors (e.g. empathy for students) and mentees, and a space for integration. Fragilities were time management for group meetings, initial themes or triggers at the start of the meetings, and sometimes difficult integration between group members.

A systematic review on mentoring programs from a global perspective are presented on **Table 1**.

Main goals: • Professional development. • Emotional well-being. • Psychosocial support. • Exposure to specific fields of medicine.
Strategies for pairing mentors and mentees: • Medical school faculty or physicians and students. • Junior to more senior medical students. • Combination of peers and faculty.
Type of meetings: • One-on-one meetings. • Group mentorship. • And less frequently remote meeting.
Students/mentees perceived benefits: • Social/personal support. • Professional development. • Advice on career. • Advice/help on choosing a field. • Increased relationship and technical skills. • To better understand clinical culture. • Opportunities for research. • Enhanced self-confidence. • Improved well-being. • Possibility of scientific publications. • Better grades. • Improved skills to prepare for exams. • Better satisfaction with rotations.
Mentors perceived benefits: • Relationship with students and next generation of physicians. • To be able to provide support. • Opportunity to become a better teacher and to improve interpersonal skills. • To stay up to date on the profession. • To be able to support a career. • To improve his/hers CV (Curriculum Vitae). • To help students build confidence.

Table 1.
A global perspective on mentoring in medical school [21].

A mentoring program can be implemented in different ways and many aspects should be considered when doing so. How should the mentor and the mentee be matched? Should it be random or based on certain characteristics of the mentee, like personal interests, career goals and so on? Who should the mentor be (staff physicians, peers) and how should he/she be recruited (volunteer basis, invitation basis)? Should the mentor have special training? What are the program goals (career development, scholarly activities, provide psychosocial support, etc)? What is the mentee-mentor ratio? Taking all this into consideration might help jump start the program [23, 25].

Mentoring can be a way to develop skills and help students manage personal and emotional challenges related to work, uncertainty and changes. There are also other programs that help develop these skills such as coaching training [26]. According to the authors this model has been used at the Imperial College (London) and Harvard Medical School "to enhance self-directed learning approaches and person-centered conversations with patients" and "emphasizes the value of setting personalized goals, exploring the wider context such as barriers and enablers, identifying options and planning next steps" (p. 1308).

2.2 Emotional regulation

Emotional Regulation is the ability to respond to emotions in an adaptative way, and includes awareness, clarity and acceptance of emotions. It is defined as "the process by which individuals influence which emotions they have, when they have them, and how they experience and express these emotions" [27] (p. 275).

Medical students and physicians are frequently exposed to situations that arouse intense negative (e.g. death, patient suffering) and positive emotions (e.g. empathy). A study with medical students [28] explored emotions (e.g. shock, anger, stress) elicited by critical incidents (e.g. patient suffering, patient dying, interaction with doctors) and how students used emotion regulation strategies. Examples of emotion regulation strategies included inaction (doing and saying nothing), trying to comfort the patient, denial, focusing on a task to avoid the emotion, reappraisal, and distancing from the situation. Reports of negative incidents were more frequent (e.g. suboptimal patient care, mistreatment) as were negative emotions (e.g. shock when facing a patient in a serious condition). Suppressing emotions is a common yet maladaptive strategy. Although it may be "a pragmatic short-term survival strategy, the long-term consequences - for doctors, for patients, and for the wider healthcare system – are potentially grave" (p. 8).

Teaching or training emotional regulation is a well-known practice to help enhance students and professionals' motivation and well-being [29]. There are several programs to improve emotional regulation, such as the Adaptive Coping with Emotions (ACE) Model, the Affect Regulation Training (ART) [30] and the DRT Skills Training Manual [31].

One strategy to help dealing with difficult emotions is TIP (Temperature, Intense exercise, and Paced breathing). One way of using temperature when dealing with difficult emotions is submerging the face in a bowl of ice-cold water to help calming down fast. Dispending high levels of energy in an intense bout of exercise has the same effect. Paced Breathing is another important mechanism to calm down and could be done almost everywhere: breathing deep into the belly and then slowly exhaling can have a calming effect (important to remember to exhale slower than inhale) [31].

Training emotional regulation is something that may be done in academic contexts with reported benefits [32]. A Social and Emotional Learning program with adolescents showed improvements in communication, decision making, problem-solving skills, emotional regulation, and resilience [33]. Emotional regulation was also studied with nurses. Donoso [29] concluded that nurses with higher emotional regulation had higher motivation to work and reported higher well-being at home when facing high emotional demands. Another study with physicians and residents showed that higher levels of self-regulating abilities are associated with higher levels of psychological well-being, suggesting that nurturing self-regulation skills could be a way to help residents and physicians to deal with the demands of their medical profession [34].

Emotional regulation is necessary during medical education, since it impacts clinical reasoning: "positive emotions in medical students are associated with a reduction in cognitive biases and more precise approaches to clinical reasoning. In contrast, anxiety and stress are associated with impaired working memory and immediate recall, subtle changes in clinical reasoning, and impaired technical and clinical functioning" [35] (p. 6).

Although emotional regulation training is a necessary and promising area, more research in academic contexts, like medical schools, are necessary.

2.3 Communication skills

Effective communication skills should be a core component for all healthcare professionals training. Several organizations, like the World Health Organization [36] emphasize good communication as a fundamental skill in order to offer good quality healthcare. Physicians should be able to stablish good quality relationship with patients and families to effectively gather relevant information (e.g. to aid diagnosis), to provide information concerning treatment option and adherence, and general interactional skills, like empathy, professional etiquette, and time management [37–39]. They also need to provide team-based work, advocated by healthcare systems in several countries [40–42].

- The C-L-A-S-S Protocol includes five core components for the medical interview: Context (setting), Listening skills, Acknowledge (validate, explore and address emotions and concerns), Strategy (propose a plan that the patient understands), and Summary (provide a summary and clarify the conversation to make sure the patient really understood)
- The S-P-I-K-E-S Protocol for breaking bad news includes: S (setting up the conversation in a quiet and private area), P (perception of the patients understanding of the situation), I (invitation to discuss the problem according to what the patient wants to know about the situation), K (knowledge means explaining the facts in a way that the patient will understand), E (emotions, that include to be empathic and supportive and to deal with the emotions as they arise), S (strategy and summary, that means to decide and clarify the best treatment plan, and to summarize the whole conversation, being prepared to answer tough questions).
- The C-O-N-E-S Protocol may be used to disclose a medical error, a sudden deterioration in the patient's condition and when talking to a family about a sudden death. C (context), O (opening shot, to alert the patient or the family about the importance of what is about to be discussed), N (narrative approach explaining the chronological sequence of events, E (emotions, using empathy to address strong emotions), S (strategy and summary, making plans to follow-up).
- The E-V-E Protocol includes three elements to be used when strong emotions occur: E (explore and identify the emotion), V (validate the emotion), and E (empathic response).

Table 2.
Examples of protocols used in medical practice [43, 44].

Sanson-Fisher et al. [39] reviewed studies about the quality of teaching communication skills to undergraduate medical students. Although they included 243 publications considered relevant, 63% of the studies were descriptive, followed by measurement studies (22%). Only 15% were intervention studies, the kind most needed "to ensure communication skills training can effectively improve interactions between clinicians and patients" (p. 1).

Examples of protocols available for different situations in clinical practice are available on **Table 2**.

3. Conclusion

A physician must be prepared to communicate well with patients, including children, adolescents, and families, people from different cultural backgrounds, and healthcare teams. Gathering and sharing information, discussing sensitive topics, breaking bad news, discussing errors, and making shared decisions are tasks inherent to the practice of medicine and must be trained during medical education. Besides technical competence, the practice of medicine also requires learning to take good care of oneself, physically and mentally. Even attending a medical school that teaches beyond cognitive and technical skills, offering good role models, emphasizing the teaching/learning of communication skills, some students will need extra help (e.g. time management, study skills), that must include mental health services for those in need.

Author details

Eduardo Miyazaki[1*], Giovanna Miyazaki[2] and M. Cristina Miyazaki[1]

1 FAMERP Medical School, São José do Rio Preto, SP, Brazil

2 Hospital de Base, São José do Rio Preto, SP, Brazil

*Address all correspondence to: esmiya@gmail.com

References

[1] Sangeetha V, Mamatha A, Vaneeta M, Beena K. Artificial intelligence in medical and healthcare service: Applications and challenges. In: Djakeli K, editor. Modern Healthcare Marketing in the Digital Era. Hershey: IGI Global; 2024. pp. 116-130. DOI: 10.4018/979-8-3693-0679-6.ch007

[2] Schukow C, Smith SC, Landgrebe E, Parasuraman S, Folaranmi OO, Paner GP, et al. Applications of ChatGPT in routine diagnostic pathology: Promises, pitfalls, and potential future directions. Advances in Anatomic Pathology. 2024;**31**(1):15-21. DOI: 10.1097/PAP.0000000000000406

[3] Huang CL. Under recognition and undertreatment of stress-related psychiatric disorders in physicians: Determinants, challenges, and the impact of the COVID-19 pandemic. World Journal of Psychiatry. 2023;**13**(4):131-140. DOI: 10.5498/wjp.v13.i4.131

[4] Mata DA, Ramos MA, Bansal N, Khan R, Guille C, Di Angelantonio E, et al. Prevalence of depression and depressive symptoms among resident physicians: A systematic review and meta-analysis. Journal of the American Medical Association. 2015;**314**(22):2373-2383. DOI: 10.1001/jama.2015.15845

[5] Harvey SB, Epstein RM, Glozier N, Petrie K, Strudwick J, Gayed A, et al. Mental illness, and suicide among physicians. The Lancet. 2021;**398**: 920-930. DOI: 10.1016/ SO140-6736(21)01596-8

[6] Mihailescu M, Neiterman E. A scoping review of the literature on the current mental health status of physicians and physicians-in-training in North America. BMC Public Health. 2019;**19**:1363. DOI: 10.1186/ s12889-019-7661-9

[7] Chutiyami M, Cheong AMY, Salihu D, Bello UM, Ndwiga D, Maharaj R, et al. COVID-19 pandemic and overall mental health of healthcare professionals globally: A meta-review of systematic reviews. Frontiers in Psychiatry. 2022;**12**:804525. DOI: 10.3389/ fpsyt.2021.804525

[8] Wu T, Jia X, Shi H, Niu J, Yin X, Xie J, et al. Prevalence of mental health problems during the COVID-19 pandemic: A systematic review and meta-analysis. Journal of Affective Disorders. 2021;**281**:91-98. DOI: 10.1016/j.jad.2020.11.117

[9] Ghahramani A, de Courten M, Prokofieva M. The potential of social media in health promotion beyond creating awareness: An integrative review. BMC Public Health. 2022;**22**(1):2402. DOI: 10.1186/ s12889-022-14885-0

[10] Wege N, Muth T, Li J, Angerer P. Mental health among currently enrolled medical students in Germany. Public Health. 2016;**132**:92-100. DOI: 10.1016/j. puhe.2015.12.014

[11] Ruitenburg MM, Frings-Dresen MH, Sluiter JK. The prevalence of common mental disorders among hospital physicians and their association with self-reported work ability: A cross-sectional study. BMC Health Services Research. 2012;**12**:292-298. DOI: 10.1186/1472-6963-12-292

[12] American Psychiatric Association (APA). Manual Diagnóstico e Estatístico de Transtornos Mentais – DSM-5-TR: Texto Revisado. Porto Alegre: Artmed; 2023

[13] Anderson DM, Diris R, Montizaan R, Rees DI. The effects of becoming a

physician on prescription drug use and mental health treatment. Journal of Health Economics. 2023;**91**:102774. DOI: 10.1016/j.jhealeco.2023.102774

[14] Wallace JE. Mental health and stigma in the medical profession. Health. 2012;**16**(1):3-18. DOI: 10.1177/1363459310371080

[15] Hussenoeder FS, Bodendieck E, Conrad I, Jung F, Riedel-Heller SG. Burnout and work-life balance among physicians: The role of migration background. Journal of Occupational Medicine and Toxicology. 2021;**16**(1):28. DOI: 10.1186/s12995-021-00318-y

[16] Macaron MM, Segun-Omosehin OA, Matar RH, Beran A, Nakanishi H, Than CA, et al. A systematic review and meta-analysis on burnout in physicians during the COVID-19 pandemic: A hidden healthcare crisis. Frontiers in Psychiatry. 2023;**13**:1071397. DOI: 10.3389/fpsyt.2022.1071397

[17] Taranu SM, Ilie AC, Turcu AM, Stefaniu R, Sandu IA, Pislaru AI, et al. Factors associated with burnout in healthcare professionals. IJEnvH. 2022;**19**(22):14701. DOI: 10.3390/ijerph192214701

[18] Braquehais MD, Vargas-Cáceres S. Psychiatric issues among health professionals. The Medical Clinics of North America. 2023;**107**(1):131-142. DOI: 10.1016/j.mcna.2022.04.004

[19] Alves SA, Sinval J, Lucas Neto L, Marôco J, Ferreira AG, Oliveira P. Burnout and dropout intention in medical students: The protective role of academic engagement. BMC Medical Education. 2022;**22**(1):1-11. DOI: 10.1186/s12909-021-03094-9

[20] Aziz A, Mahboob U, Sethi A. What problems make students struggle during their undergraduate medical education? A qualitative exploratory study. Pakistan Journal of Medical Science. 2020;**36**(5):1020-1024. DOI: 10.12669/pjms.36.5.2267

[21] Atlas AM, Seltzer ES, Watters A, Riley B, Chan T. A global perspective of mentorship in medical schools: Systematic review from 2014 to 2019. Medical Science Education. 2021;**31**(2):969-977. DOI: 10.1007/s40670-021-01252-8

[22] Fornari A, Murray TS, Menzin AW, Woo VA, Clifton M, Lombardi M, et al. Mentoring program design and implementation in new medical schools. Medical Education Online. 2014;**19**(1): 24570. DOI: 10.3402/meo.v19.24570

[23] Silva EFSF, Miyazaki MCOS. Implementation of mentoring in a medical school – Mentors and students' perceptions. REBEM. 2022;**46**(1):e030. DOI: 10.1590/1981-5271v46.1-20200501.ing

[24] Johnson WB. On Being a Mentor. A Guide for Higher Education Faculty. 2nd ed. New York: Routledge; 2016

[25] Joe MB, Cusano A, Leckie J, Czuczman N, Exner K, Yong H, et al. Mentorship programs in residency: A scoping review. Journal of Graduate Medical Education. 2023;**15**(2):190-200. DOI: 10.4300/JGME-D-22-00415.1

[26] Maini A, Saravanan Y, Singh TA, Fyfe M. Coaching skills for medical education in a VUCA world. Medical Teacher. 2020;**42**(11):1308-1309. DOI: 10.1080/0142159X.2020.1788713

[27] Gross JJ. The emerging field of emotion regulation: An integrative review. Review of General Psychology. 1998;**2**(3):271-299. DOI: 10.1037/1089-2680.2.3.271

[28] Doulougeri K, Panagopoulou E, Montgomery A. (How) do medical students regulate their emotions? BMC Medical Education. 2016;**16**(1):312. DOI: 10.1186/s12909-016-0832-9

[29] Donoso LMB, Demerouti E, Hernandez EG, Moreno-Jimenez B, Cobo IC. Positive benefits of caring on nurses' motivation and well-being: A diary study about the role of emotional regulation abilities at work. International Journal of Nursing Studies. 2015;**52**(4):804-816. DOI: 10.1016/j.ijnurstu.2015.01.002

[30] Buruck G, Dörfel D, Kugler J, Brom SS. Enhancing well-being at work: The role of emotion regulation skills as personal resources. Journal of Occupational Health Psychology. 2016;**21**(4):480-493. DOI: 10.1037/ocp0000023

[31] Linehan M. DBT Skills training manual. New York: Guilford; 2014

[32] Hoffmann JD, Brackett MA, Bailey CS, Willner CJ. Teaching emotion regulation in schools: Translating research into practice with the RULER approach to social and emotional learning. Emotion. 2020;**20**(1):105-109. DOI: 10.1037/emo0000649

[33] Green AL, Ferrante S, Boaz TL, Kutash K, Wheeldon RB. Social and emotional learning during early adolescence: Effectiveness of a classroom-based SEL program for middle school students. Psychology in the Schools. 2021;**58**(6):1056-1069. DOI: 10.1002/pits.22487

[34] Simon CR, Durand-Bush N. Differences in psychological and affective well-being between physicians and resident physicians: Does high and low self-regulation capacity matter? Psychology Well-Being. 2014;**4**:1-19. DOI: 10.1186/s13612-014-0019-2

[35] Toufan N, Omid A, Haghani F. The double-edged sword of emotions in medical education: A scoping review. Journal of Education Health Promotion. 2023;**12**:52. DOI: 10.4103/jehp.jehp_644_21

[36] World Health Organization – WHO. Global Strategy on Human Resources for Health: Workforce 2030. [Internet] 2016. 2016. Available from: https://www.who.int/hrh/resources/global_strategy_workforce2030_14_print.pdf?ua=1

[37] Choudhary A, Gupta V. Teaching communications skills to medical students: Introducing the fine art of medical practice. IJBAR. 2015, 2015;**5**(Suppl):S41-S44. DOI: 10.4103/2229-516X.162273

[38] Ruiz de Azua S, Ozamiz-Etxebarria N, Ortiz-Jauregui MA, Gonzalez-Pinto A. Communicative and social skills among medical students in Spain: A descriptive analysis. IJEnvH. 2020;**17**(4):1408. DOI: 10.3390/ijerph17041408

[39] Sanson-Fisher R, Hobden B, Waller A, Dodd N, Boyd L. Methodological quality of teaching communication skills to undergraduate medical students: A mapping review. BMC Medical Education. 2018;**8**(1):151. DOI: 10.1186/s12909-018-1265-4

[40] Lutfiyya MN, Chang LF, McGrath C, Dana C, Lipsky MS. The state of the science of interprofessional collaborative practice: A scoping review of the patient health-related outcomes based on literature published between 2010 and 2018. PLoS One. 2019;**14**(6):e0218578. DOI: 10.1371/journal.pone.0218578

[41] Nguyen KH, Chien AT, Meyers DJ, Li Z, Singer SJ, Rosenthal MB. Team-based primary care practice transformation initiative and

changes in patient experience and recommended cancer screening rates. Inquiry. 2020;**57**:1-8. DOI: 10.1177/0046958020952911

[42] Robiner WN, Hong BA, Ward W. Psychologists' contributions to medical education and Interprofessional education in medical schools. Journal of Clinical Psychology in Medical Settings. 2020;**28**(4):666-678. DOI: 10.1007/s10880-020-09730-8

[43] MD Anderson Cancer Center. The Complete Guide to Communication Skills in Clinical Practice [Internet]. 2014. Available from: https://www.mdanderson.org

[44] Baile WF, Buckman R, Lenzi R, Glober G, Beale EA, Kudelka AP. SPIKES-A six-step protocol for delivering bad news: Application to the patient with cancer. The Oncologist. 2000;**5**(4):302-311. DOI: 10.1634/theoncologist.5-4-302

Section 2

Professionalism in Medical Education

Chapter 3

Professional Behavior in Medical Practice

Vida Seifouri

Abstract

Nowadays, ethical and behavioral responsibilities have been expanded in a range of individual-personal responsibilities to personal-occupational responsibilities. Professional behavior is one of the basic issues in human societies. If a comprehensive definition of ethical principles is provided, professionals in any job can decide what behavior is reasonable and unreasonable and which action is ethical and which is unethical. In the medical community, the discussion of behavior has a special place due to the importance of the medical profession, so medical ethics has a very serious and extensive scientific discussion. If the benefits of observing professional behavior are more comprehensive, the level of commitment to its principles is of a higher degree, and the more reasonable the restrictions imposed due to the principles of professional behavior, the stronger the adherence to it. In this chapter, the definition, importance, characteristics of professional behavior in medicine and its behavioral areas, as well as the methods of teaching professional behavior and its evaluation criteria are discussed. Finally, general guidelines for medical professional behavior are provided.

Keywords: professional behavior, professionalism, medical commitment, medical ethics, professional behavior training

1. Introduction

Professionalism is not a new concept and has existed throughout the history of medicine in the form of medical oaths. What makes the doctor-patient relationship effective and is necessary for the doctor's success in diagnosing, treating, and providing preventive services is the patient's trust in the doctor. What makes medicine a sacred and valuable profession is the trust that the society has in the servants of this profession. Trusting that the employees of this profession have set their main goal to ensure people's health and prioritize it over their own interests and commit to this sacred goal in the form of an oath.

The characteristics of a profession are:

1. Working in a profession generally requires specialized knowledge or skills.

2. The society grants special privileges to the members of the profession.

3. The society expects them to put the interests of the society before their own interests in providing social services [1].

The society has given the right to the health service system to decide and implement what it considers appropriate regarding the provision of health services to the patients and the society and to evaluate the correctness of the performance of its members and the processes of the health system. In order to provide their services, doctors have the privilege to ask patients for confidential information, examine the patient's naked body, and perform procedures on the patient's body. Of course, in return for granting this right, he expects this profession to prioritize the interests of society over all its goals and to guarantee the quality of services by training and monitoring the professional performance of its members [2]. Therefore, the health system as well as the individual members of the medical profession are committed to make their decisions and actions that serve the health of patients and prioritize the patient's interests over their own interests.

2. Characteristics of professional behavior in medicine

Professionalism is adherence to obligations, and it is one of the most important capabilities that every medical student must acquire and demonstrate in practice and behavior. The characteristics of a person that is a manifestation of professionalism in professional behavior are:

- *Altruism*: The doctor is obliged to seek the best interests of the patients.
- *Professional excellence*: A doctor is committed to learning medical science and skills throughout his professional life.
- *Conscientiousness (obligation)*: The doctor must be committed to serving in his profession and perform his duties completely and on time.
- *Truth and honor*: The doctor must be committed to observing fairness, honesty, and correctness in his interactions with patients and his profession.
- *Respect for others*: The doctor is obliged to respect the patients and their families, other doctors, and other team members, medical students, assistants, and fellows.
- *Justice*: The doctor is obliged to facilitate the fair provision of services and eliminate discrimination in the provision of services [3, 4].

Examples of each of the components of professional behavior:

2.1 Altruism

- Prioritizing the patient's interests over his own interests.
- Showing attention to the patient's wishes.
- Spending time and patience to explain the information to the patient.

- Spending time and patience to comfort a critical patient.
- Trying to reduce the suffering and pain of the patient in all possible ways.
- Compassionately listening to the patient's concerns.
- Participation in local and national professional organizations.
- Offering help to other team members volunteering to do the work of another person who cannot do his work.
- Providing to others with their knowledge and skills.

2.2 Professional excellence

- Active search for feedbacks.
- Modifying one's behavior or performance based on the provided feedback.
- A critical attitude toward oneself and the ability to identify areas of one's ability and knowledge that need improvement.
- Knowing his limitations and getting help from others in cases where his knowledge and skills are not enough.
- Adaptability to changing conditions.
- Assessing own physical, mental, and spiritual health.
- Feeling responsible for your retraining.
- Participation in rounds, seminars, and other educational activities.
- Study based on the cases of patients who refer to him.

2.3 Conscientiousness (obligation)

- Arriving on time.
- Being reliable.
- Follow the supervisor.
- Complete the assigned duties completely and on time.
- Responding to letters, summons (pages), telephones, and emails in a timely manner.
- Compliance with rules and regulations.

- Appropriate cooperation in teamwork.
- Performing duties and being available on call.
- Accurate and complete report of the care that is done for the patient.
- Correct and complete transfer of patient care responsibility.
- Notifying others when he cannot be present to perform the duty and making sure that there is a substitute for him.
- Completing the care of patients before discharging them.
- Reporting medical errors to the team or supervisor.
- Declaration of conflict of interest to the team or supervisor.
- Identifying and reporting errors and inappropriate behavior of colleagues by avoiding unfairly discrediting their reputation.
- Participation in professional self-monitoring activities.
- Avoiding drug and alcohol abuse.
- Providing effective criticism instead of complaining.

2.4 Truth and honor

- Honest behavior: truthfulness, fairness, to be frank, keeping the promise resolving disputes in a way that respects the dignity of the other party.
- Proper behavior of medical dignity, whether in behavior, speech, or the way of dressing and grooming.
- Being honest with patients and avoiding exaggerating your capabilities.
- Encouraging the successes of your colleagues in public gatherings.
- Commenting only on the topics that are in his area of expertise.
- Nonparticipation in cheating (giving and taking) in exams.
- Accepting responsibility for your work.
- Avoid using unfair methods to improve your academic position.
- Not participating in exploitative relationships with colleagues, students, patients, or their families in order to gain material, emotional, sexual, research, or educational benefits.

- Ethical conduct and honest reporting of research and proper appreciation of the participation of others in the publication of the research work.

- Avoiding plagiarism.

2.5 Respect for others

- Establishing understanding with team members.

- Maintaining the necessary privacy in occupational and educational situations.

- Introducing yourself and the team members to the patient and his family.

- Addressing the patient in an appropriate way.

- Using terms that can be understood by the patient in talking with the patient.

- Respecting and preserving the human dignity of patients and their families, whether in their presence or in their absence, in discussions with other members of the treatment team.

- Respecting the patient's right to individual autonomy by providing information about treatment choices to them or their guardians.

- Providing advice to the patient's family or legal guardian, when he lacks decision-making capacity.

- Respecting the confidentiality and privacy of the patient.

- Maintaining the necessary privacy in relation to the patient.

- Good and appropriate communication with subordinate students in the educational environment.

- Good and appropriate communication with professors in the educational environment.

- Good and proper communication with the staff of other health-related professions.

- Showing tolerance and patience in front of a range of behaviors and opinions.

- Nondiscrimination in your interactions with others based on things such as age, race, skin color, race, political opinions, marital status, physical and mental disabilities, gender, sexual orientation (homosexual or nonhomosexual), or criminal convictions.

2.6 Commitment to social justice

- Equitable distribution of health-care resources.

- Medicine based on cost-effectiveness.
- Taking care of health service resources.

3. Four areas of professional behavior

The behaviors that doctors may show are in a spectrum from ideal behavior to ugly behavior. Below are examples of behaviors that fall into each of these areas:

3.1 Ideal behavior

- Forgiving toward colleagues, patients, and patients' families.
- Altruistic toward others.
- Good-natured and flexible.
- Humility toward one's successes.
- Eager to teach students and their questions.
- Arresting patients, employees, and consultants.
- To be available and serve continuously and more than necessary.
- Quenching the anger and anxiety of patients and employees.
- Being a role model inside and outside the work environment.
- Doing the right thing only for moral reasons.

3.2 Desired/expected behavior

- Arriving on time and getting ready for work.
- Prioritizing the interests of the patient.
- Completing patient care before discharging them.
- Protecting the interests and privacy of the patient.
- Respectful treatment of patients and their families, employees, and colleagues.
- Training other team members (students, employees, and residents).
- Discussing difficult issues (treatment choices, decision-making, end of life, and telling the truth) in a kind manner with the patient, their family, and other employees.
- Open-minded acceptance of criticism from professors and staff.

3.3 Undesired behavior

- Arriving late or getting ready for work late.
- Disclosure of patients' information.
- Failure to correctly hand over responsibility for patient care.
- Saying insulting and annoying words or information.
- Accepting significant gifts from founders or pharmaceutical companies.
- Performing nonsurgical medical procedures without valid consent from the patient.
- Self-reference.
- Discrimination between students or patients based on race, gender, religion, or other objective characteristics.
- Disrespectful interaction with patients, their families, or employees.
- Failure to properly mention the names and efforts of others when their work has been used for education or research.
- Failure to implement or respond appropriately to the professorate's recommendations or teachings.
- Changing programs in your favor.
- Using altruism as an excuse to avoid other duties.

3.4 Ugly behavior

- Abandoning the patient.
- Unavailability during on call.
- Repeated lying, cheating, or stealing.
- Substance abuse or addiction.
- Not learning from past mistakes.
- Showing or broadcasting erotic photos and other annoying things in the work environment.
- Creating a danger that is very threatening to the health of patients or employees.

- Verbal or physical insults to patients, their families, or employees.
- Distortion in medical reports or research data.
- Theft of medicine or medical devices.
- Sexual assault on patients or colleagues.

4. Why is professional behavior important, and why should it be taught?

Today, some believe that doctors are less altruistic than in the past, and this has led to a decrease in trust in the profession. There are also threats and factors that make us pay more attention to the category of professional behavior than before. These factors and threats can be divided into two categories, internal and external. Some of the internal factors and threats of professional behavior are: abuse of power, pride, greed, providing false information (lies and fraud), lack of conscientiousness, and conflict of interests. Inadequate knowledge and expertise can also threaten the professional behavior of the doctor [5].

Among the external factors and threats to professional behavior and commitment, the following can be mentioned: Rapid growth of medical knowledge and skills, increasing media attention to health-care issues, change in the philosophy of patient care, multidisciplinary teamwork in health care, the changes made in the attitude of doctors, pressures from colleagues, and commercial and speculative view of health.

Another concern that has been created recently is the professional behavior of the doctor in the virtual space and social networks, because some doctors consider virtual space to be different from the real space and may have misbehaviors in virtual space that distorts people's trust in the profession [6].

On the other hand, studies have shown that unfavorable practices in medicine are more caused by unprofessional behaviors than by the lack of knowledge or skills of doctors.

In a review study [7], it was shown that there is a relationship between unprofessional behavior and adverse outcomes such as patient endangerment, patient dissatisfaction, and medical malpractice lawsuits. And there are also various studies that show that students who had unprofessional behaviors during their studies continued this trend in their future performance as doctors [8]. In short, we conclude from this section that today more than in the past, paying attention to professional behavior in educational programs is important and should be taught.

5. What methods and approaches are not there for training professional commitment?

It is now clear that unprofessional behavior cannot be controlled through disciplinary measures and codes of ethics alone. Rather, active training programs should be formulated for the development of professional behavior and commitment.

Of course, there were discussions in the past on whether it is possible to teach professional behavior and commitment at all. Considering the large amount of evidence available, the inclusion of professional behavior in competency frameworks and curricula in medical education is in no doubt. What is being discussed is the correct method of teaching and evaluating professional behavior and also acknowledging this point that due to multifaceted and context-dependent professional behavior, teaching it is not easy compared to teaching medical knowledge and skills. In this section, we discuss different methods, approaches, and opinions regarding professional behavior training. The meaning of education is its more general concept, not a teaching method [9].

6. Professional behavior training: explicit or implicit?

In the past, there was a debate on whether professional behavior should be explicitly taught or implicitly taught [10]. But it seems that nowadays, the approach is to use both types of education. First, it is better to clarify a concept:

Three levels or three types of curriculum can be imagined in medical schools.

1. The declared curriculum or the written program: it is designed by the faculty or the ministry and is announced for implementation.

2. The taught curriculum: it is what happens in practice.

3. Learned curriculum: it is what students do not learn. Students do not just learn from the taught curriculum; they learn things that the faculty did not intend to teach them. Experts call this type of curriculum as hidden curriculum.

Therefore, the hidden curriculum is the learning that the faculty did not intend to teach, but the students have learned during their education. Skiles simply states that in the hidden curriculum, students learn something that comes from the difference between our behavior and speech (teachers, managers, etc.) [11]. Therefore, for professional behavior training to be effective, both explicit training and implicit training are necessary in the formal curriculum. Of course, it is important to mention that the professional identity is formed during the course of medical education and the educational intervention should be integrated into the entire training course. Therefore, it is necessary for all lecturers and professors to transfer this concept and improve its application in decisions that have an active and effective clinical role [12]. Integrated education is not discussed in this chapter, and only effective educational methods are examined.

7. Teaching professional behavior in the formal curriculum

Professional behavior has a cognitive dimension or basis, and it can be done directly using him taught different methods. First, it should be ensured that the learners understand the nature of professional behavior, the reasons and why to observe it, and its features and examples. The goal is for them to reach a common language of concepts and examples of professional behavior. In the basic cognitive training of professional behavior, a variety of common methods can be used, such as interactive lectures, case-based learning, teaching in small groups, e-learning, and so forth. [11]. But if the training is only limited to defining professional behavior and listing a series of characteristics and behaviors that follow from it, then only theoretical knowledge has been provided to the learners, and as a result, the impact of the provided training will be much less. Therefore, to internalize those traits and values, other educational methods are needed.

7.1 Reflection

Experiential learning is a process that a person learns through experiencing. However, experience alone is not enough for effective learning. Experience must be integrated into one's existing knowledge structure and interpreted accordingly in order to generate new knowledge or expand existing knowledge. Reflection is critical to this active learning process [13].

Reflection is "a conscious examination of the ideas, feelings, meaning, and meaning of learning experiences." There are different models and theories in the field of reflection.

But the reflection process can be simply summarized in these three steps:

1. Doing (gaining experience).

2. Evaluation and analysis of that experience.

3. Planning for future performance.

These steps continue cyclically. Reflection is used for various purposes, but in the case of professional behavior, it is at the heart of many educational programs [14]. Reflection transforms experience into greater understanding and makes a person reach higher levels of learning. Reflection helps students to integrate theoretical knowledge and knowledge gained from experience and can plan to improve their future performance.

In the training of professional behavior, critical incident report and narration is used as a stimulus for formal reflection. However, during clinical encounters, depending on the situation and event that happens to the learners, the professor and the tutor can encourage the learner to think and guide him to achieve the educational result hidden in the situation. Critical incidents are difficult situations that students experience or unexpected consequences that result from individual student performance. These events are usually associated with feelings such as anger, frustration, excitement, and so on.

In various studies, the effectiveness of reflection in professional behavior training has been investigated, and reflection has been reported as one of the main and effective methods in the professional behavior training program [15].

7.2 Other specified training methods of professional behavior

There are other ways to teach professional behavior that we only mention their titles below.

- (Role-playing) performance

- Use of film

- Simulation-based training

- Journal club
- Team-based learning
- Learning based on problem solving
- Educational folder.

7.3 Implicit training of professional behavior

7.3.1 Role modeling

In a qualitative study using the grounded theory method, surgical assistants stated that they learn professional behavior through the following sources and methods:

- Personal values and family upbringing.
- Behavior patterns.
- The structure of the surgical residency course.
- And their formal training with role models.

For centuries, behavioral patterns have been the responsibility of transmitting medical attitudes and values. Undoubtedly, behavior patterns play an important role in the formation of students' professional personality [16].

Now the question that arises is who are role models? In response, it should be said that all professors play the role of models for learners to some extent. Is this a positive thing?

The answer must be absolutely no! Because negative behavior patterns are abundant in the university and hospital environment and students may imitate their negative behaviors.

Therefore, there is a need for positive behavior patterns in educational environments. These patterns have a series of characteristics that Passi et al. [17] classified into three categories in the BEME systematic review guide number 27, which can be seen in **Table 1**.

Students are more influenced by professors' behavior than their words. Therefore, the ideal would be that the words of teachers are the same as their behavior (good words, good deeds). Some believe that for role models to be more effective, they need to know what behavior or role they are modeling. Or in other words, they should know what kind of behavior is modeled on them by the students. This points to the importance of empowering faculty members, which we will discuss in the relevant section.

It seems that students are even more influenced by negative behavioral patterns than by positive behavioral patterns [13]. The recommendation is to remove such patterns from the educational environment if possible, and if this is not possible, we should inform the students and give them feedback so that they recognize the negative behavior patterns and use it as an effective educational experience.

Category	Examples
Clinical qualification	High level of knowledge and clinical skills Patient-centered approach Human behaviors such as empathy, respect, and compassion
Teaching skills	Giving relaxation to learners Creating a positive and supportive educational environment Designing and using special teaching methods Committed to the growth of learners Providing the opportunity for students to interact with patients at the bedside Conscious pivot pattern
Personal characteristics	Effective interpersonal skills Having a positive attitude and perspective Honesty Leadership skills Committed to excellence Honest, polite, enthusiastic, and inspiring to students

Table 1.
Characteristics of a good role model.

In general, model-oriented is a very effective method for creating professional identity in students, but it is not enough in any way. In the past, professors had a lot of interaction with students and there were fewer challenges for professional performance, but nowadays, the contact between professor and student of general medicine course has decreased and there are many obstacles for professional performance.

Therefore, there is a need for other methods to teach professional behavior, some of which we mentioned. An appropriate balance must be struck between explicit and implicit teaching of professional behavior [18]. The next important point is the empowerment of faculty members, because for the success and effectiveness of any educational program, it is necessary to empower faculty members. First, professors should be familiar with the definition, nature, importance, and components of professional behavior and commitment (cognitive basis (and then learn the appropriate methods of teaching and evaluating it.

7.3.2 Empowerment

To advance each of the goals of improving professional behavior, it is necessary to increase human capital and bring faculty members together. This can be delegated to the center for studies and education development of the university. One of the most important goals of the center for the study and development of medical education in universities is to design, implement, and evaluate programs to create, maintain, develop, and improve the capabilities and strengthen the scientific power and practical skills of professors in order to improve the quality of education and teaching of the university to meet the changing needs of the societies, health systems, and educational needs of its members [3].

As stated, the behavior and performance of professors can play a key role in shaping the professional behavior of students. One of the most important functions of professors is how to communicate with patients. Doctor's interaction with the patient is one of the necessities of the medical profession, and communication with the patient is a basic clinical skill and the most important characteristic required for professors and doctors.

On the one hand, the professors will be responsible for the correct transmission of scientific concepts, and on the other hand, they will be the practical and human model of moral values in the work environment [2]. Professional behavior can be done through the exemplary role of professors in the educational environment in an inconspicuous way that should be taught to students through performance.

8. Evaluation of medical professional behavior

Professional medical behavior is one of the most important competencies that should be studied in medical students. Evaluation of professional behavior helps us to know the current situation and know where we are going so that we can help it to grow and excel.

The assessment of this competence can be implemented at different stages. The most ideal situation is for it to take place at the beginning of entering the university, but this issue is not applicable in practice and we still do not have a suitable tool for this evaluation. The content of professional behavior assessment includes both personality and performance of people and does not only include a checklist of personal and behavioral characteristics.

Another important point is that according to the stages of change and progress of education, the evaluation should be individualized and should be done according to the strategies of each educational level [19]. For example, knowledge should be evaluated for lower level students, and performance should be checked for higher levels. The last point is that effective evaluation should be in two ways: providing feedback or adding a score and feedback should be considered constructive and not punitive.

8.1 Criteria for evaluating medical professional behavior

In the discussion of evaluating the professional behavior of doctors, two categories of skills are mentioned:

1. Cognitive skills include gathering information, diagnosis, management, performing procedures, and application of technology.

2. Noncognitive skills include:

    - Communication (language, sympathy, integrity, and empathy).

    - Interaction (responsibility, respect, and performance of duties).

    - Continuous improvement (recognizing limitations and motivating progress).

In the literature review, long lists of competencies were examined as criteria for professional behavior, which include the following:

Having professional relationships; appropriate behavior with other people; righteousness and honesty; empathy; the lack of influence of the doctor's bad mood on the patient's treatment; matching with the patient's level of understanding; having interest in the patient; flexibility; friendliness; commitment to maintaining the progressive flow of medical progress and excellence (pursuing life-long knowledge acquisition); effective patient communication; respect for patients' autonomy; teamwork; communication skills; respect; responsibility; transferring knowledge and skills to the next generation and serving the society and the general public; informed consent; altruism,;spending time to care for the patient despite the risks; identifying mistakes; being a person of scientific research and publication; efforts to increase the quality of care, honor, and punctuality; paying attention to the culture, age, gender, and disabilities of the patients and establishing a suitable verbal relationship with them; being humble, polite, and well-spoken; being a good listener; time management; having a supportive attitude; complete and accurate documentation of patient care and learning activities; being self-motivated; using learning opportunities; providing constructive feedback; appropriate appearance; paying attention to the organization's goals; adapt to changes in problem-solving; critical thinking; crisis management and challenges such as having little time to implement things; social justice; talking to the patient with expressive language and friendly behavior; creating a positive learning environment; social responsibility toward being strong toward patients and accepting their mistakes and apologizing; sharing the best professional judgment; and leadership [20, 21].

8.2 Medical professional behavior measurement tools.

The most difficult step in the assessment of professional behavior is the selection of tools. Professional behavior evaluation tools are very wide such as: self-evaluation, simulation like the Objective Structured Clinical Examination (OSCE); direct supervision like multiple feedback, patient opinion, and role model evaluation (learners' evaluation of their teacher as a role model); evaluation with the help of standard patient; evaluation of professional environment (evaluation of the learning environment or the work environment and not a specific individual review); multiple choice question; and video and scenario analysis.

Among other very valuable methods, evaluation of professional behavior is a 360-degree method [1]. But the drawback of this method is that it is not used in terms of patients. Despite the fact that the core of medical professional behavior is the doctor–patient relationship and the "patient" is at the center of the doctor's philosophy of existence and professional presence, paying attention to the opinion of patients is neglected in this field.

One of the most effective ways to discover unprofessional behaviors can be the eyes and ears of patients and their families, and with this perspective, in addition to using the comprehensive opinion, colleagues, professors, and so forth in the evaluation of professionalism, also is using in the opinion of patients.

One of the practical questionnaires in evaluating medical professionalism is the professional questionnaire of the American Board of Internal Medicine [22] (ADIM) that assesses professionalism in the form of 7 areas and 36 items and provides a valuable 360-degree assessment of the hidden curriculum [23].

In order to achieve the goals of medical professionalism and the correct training of future doctors, it is necessary that the curriculum based on medical professionalism be implemented in all universities of every country and continuously evaluated and modified. According to the studies conducted in the discussion of medical professionalism in order to deepen the education of this category, it is appropriate to study the strategies of integrating professionalism in the medical education curriculum and the causes of professionalism fatigue in the medical staff and the solutions to solve it [24].

9. General guide of professional medical behavior

Today, several factors have caused the need to introduce new and updated ethical standards to activities in this field. Scientific and technological advances in methods of prevention, diagnosis, treatment, and rehabilitation of patients and other recipients of health services have led to many new situations and questions that have never been seen before in the history of medical ethics.

The emergence of new concepts such as "brain death" and "organ transplant," the possibility of diagnosing diseases and abnormalities before birth, the dramatic expansion of genetic technologies, the possibility of predicting diseases using genetic information and creating the possibility of modifying the human genome in the initial stages, and many other scientific and technological developments have led to the creation of fundamental questions in the field of end-of-life care, abortion, and manipulation of the human genome.

Establishing the "right to health" for all citizens and the moral duty of governments to provide for health-related needs has led to the creation of large and complex health systems, in which the development of medical technologies adds to this complexity every day. The creation of these large and complex health systems, with their diverse components (including the pharmaceutical industry and medical equipment, politicians and health policymakers, and managers of different levels), has changed the position of medical and related professionals from direct and individual providers of health services to people who are in the framework. The health system and interaction with other stakeholders have changed.

This change of position has also brought new ethical requirements for this group and has made the need to provide new behavioral standards to help the medical professionals to adjust their relationships with the various elements of the health system a special necessity.

The specialization and superspecialization of health services is another change that creates some special ethical requirements for medical professionals. This phenomenon requires the aforementioned group to have specific norms for interaction with other specialists, colleagues, and members of treatment teams and various governmental and nongovernmental sectors of the health system. The change in the pattern of diseases from infectious diseases to chronic diseases, the increase in the average lifespan of humans, and the aging of societies in recent decades have also led to a serious change in the way medical professionals communicate with patients, and it has resulted in many moral consequences that originated from the long continuity of communication between patients and the professionals of this profession.

The general guide to the professional behavior of medical professionals includes a set of values, norms, principles, and ethical rules that were compiled based on the principle of human dignity, and all the items in this guide have the same importance and should be considered as a set.

9.1 General assignments

- Medical professionals must refrain from doing any act that is known to be against professional ethics, that is, that causes disrespect to the medical profession or harms the public trust in doctors.

- The use of tobacco, drugs, psychotropic substances, and alcohol in clinical environments and addiction to alcohol, narcotic drugs, and psychotropic substances are among the cases of professional misconduct.

- Taking a medical oath means accepting a permanent obligation to provide diagnostic and treatment services to all people, to the best of one's ability.Medical professionals must provide health services to all referring patients regardless of any discrimination related to gender, nationality, race, ethnicity, religion, social, political and economic status, or type of disease.

- In dealing with patients, their companions and colleagues at different levels, and commenting on people, ethnicities, and social groups, it is necessary to respect the human dignity of people, social etiquette, and general politeness and avoid any act that includes insults, humiliation, and labeling.

- Medical professionals are responsible for ensuring compliance with professional ethics standards by their subordinates, including assistants, employees, and other people who are in contact with patients due to cooperation with professionals (such as office clerks), as much as possible.

- It is necessary for medical professionals to maintain their composure and calmness at all times, especially when they are angry.Those medical and allied professionals, who, for any reason, may lose control when angry, need to take preventive measures in this regard. In any case, it is necessary to refrain from any forceful and disrespectful behavior outside the framework of politeness, even in response to insults and verbal insults.

- Medical professionals should treat patients and their companions with kindness, altruism, and compassion as much as possible, and health professionals should do their best to improve their personal capacity to empathize with patients.

- It is necessary to avoid actions that involve the expression of emotions out of proportion to the situation, such as joking with other colleagues in situations where patients or patients' companions are in a state of extreme anxiety and worry (such as during cardiopulmonary resuscitation(.

- It is necessary in dealing with patients, besides physical health, other dimensions of the patient's health, including the psychological dimension (including possible concerns) and social dimension (including family and friendly relations, lifestyle, and interpersonal communication); they should take into account the spiritual dimension of the patients as well as other possible psychological and social contexts in which the disease has occurred and provide them with the necessary recommendations by mentioning the reason for the connection of such factors with the disease of people.

- It is necessary to take all the necessary and possible measures to minimize the pain and suffering of the patients. In all stages, it is necessary to use standard palliative methods, along with performing diagnostic, therapeutic, and rehabilitation interventions for patients.

- In addition to the human dignity of people during their lifetime, the body of a dead person is respected.

- It is necessary to refrain from any action that is considered as "desecration of the dead" and also from taking pictures and filming of corpses, except for legitimate reasons. Compliance with this issue is more important for those medical professionals who work in the process of autopsy of deceased people.

9.2 Providing services standard and high quality

- Medical professionals are obliged to use the maximum possible effort to provide the best health services to their patients within the limits of their legal and professional duties and available facilities.

- In cases where medical professionals realize that they do not have the necessary scientific and practical qualifications to start or continue the process of providing health services, they should use the advice of other colleagues or refer the patient to a qualified institution or professional.

- In cases where the patient's life is in serious and imminent danger due to a medical emergency, the medical professionals are obliged to do their utmost to stabilize the patient's condition at the same time or before consulting or referring the patient.

- Health care should be provided based on appropriate and up-to-date diagnostic and treatment methods available and based on scientific evidence and current medical knowledge.

- Providing any service outside of approved clinical guidelines, approved or specialized scientific references, under any title, as well as referring patients to people who claim treatment with nonscientific methods and non-reputable centers by medical professionals is prohibited. It is clear that if the safety and effectiveness of any treatment claim is proven during standard research, these cases will be considered part of modern medical science.

- Merely having a medical degree or other related professional qualifications at any stage does not justify any type of medical intervention. Medical professionals are allowed to treat patients only in the areas where they have received formal training and acquired the necessary scientific and practical skills. The authority for determining acceptable training is the organization of the medical system.

9.3 Priority of the patient's interests

- It is necessary to prioritize the interests of the patient over any other benefit (including benefits that may accrue to the family or relatives by ignoring the patient's interests) in offering any health intervention to patients (including all diagnostic and therapeutic measures).

- It is necessary to avoid imposing any unnecessary or unfounded costs on patients, in any form and title.To encourage patients to use unnecessary services, reasons such as self-defense against a possible patient complaint or benefiting a third person or institution are not justified.

- Medical professionals, in cases where they accept the responsibility of providing services to patients and other recipients of health services, are responsible for the continuation of the patient's treatment, to the extent of their ability and expertise.

- Failure to accept patients is only acceptable due to the existence of justified limitations (such as lack of time and suitable facilities or lack of sufficient technical and scientific ability).

- It is necessary for medical professionals to act based on the priority of the patient's interests in situations that may put their interests in conflict with the interests of patients (including participation in any agreement or contract).

- It is necessary to prioritize the patient's interests and medical resources in referring patients to other medical and allied professionals or para-clinical institutions, such as imaging centers, pharmacies, hospitals, laboratories, and the like; all referrals should be in the benefits of patients, according to accepted scientific standards and based on the professional competence and ability of the health service provider or the quality of the centers providing diagnostic and therapeutic services to which the patient is referred.

- Receiving and granting any rewards or points, including cash, gifts, discounts on rent or office fees, requests for cross-referrals of patients, and the like, in exchange for referring patients to other medical and allied professionals or to diagnostic and treatment centers, hospitals, laboratories, imaging centers, rehabilitation centers or medical equipment companies, pharmacies, and the like are prohibited.

- Doctors should not in applying and using diagnostic and therapeutic equipment in the office or clinic (such as echocardiography, endoscopy, electroencephalogram, electrocardiogram, etc., which are allowed in the office according to professional rules and regulations) prefer their interests over the interests of patients.

- It is necessary to refrain from accepting any type of gift from the patient and his companions that affects the professional judgment and the process of providing services to the patient. Accepting conventional gifts with little financial value (such as flowers, sweets, and certificates of appreciation given by patients) is fine. It is necessary to not accept the gift in a suitable way that does not cause resentment or embarrassment to the patients, and the reason for not accepting the gift should be explained to the patient.

- Medical professionals are obliged to act in relation to the pharmaceutical industry and medical equipment in such a way that their professional judgment and loyalty to scientific principles are not affected.

- Medical professionals should refrain from writing advertising recommendations regarding the value or usefulness or superiority of the exclusive products of companies and industries, upon the request of these companies and institutions.

- Unless the publication of research results that have been approved by an ethical committee in valid research and during which the benefits of a specific drug or product are reported.

- It is necessary for doctors to be appropriately available throughout the diagnosis and treatment period for the patients they are treating, and how to reach them or their assistants with scientific and practical qualifications to establish contact and obtain guidance in emergency situations should be provided to patients. In cases where medical professionals are out of reach for any reason, including travel and the like, it is necessary to provide the necessary arrangements to replace someone with acceptable scientific and practical qualifications. This replacement must be appropriately written and informed to the patients.

- Guiding patients from government, government-affiliated, and charitable health-care institutions to private sector (both hospitals and clinics and vice versa) for financial use by medical professionals is prohibited.

- Abandoning patients who need to receive health services, without handing over the patient to another qualified professional, for reasons such as the end of the work shift, is not acceptable in any way. It is necessary for medical professionals to ensure that the patient is not abandoned after the end of their shift and transfer the responsibility of his care to other doctors who are qualified for this.

- Proposing or establishing any personal or sexual emotional relationship with patients and their companions as long as there is a professional and therapeutic relationship with the patient is prohibited for medical professionals. Doctors are obliged to refrain from using their position as a therapist for any exploitation (such as sexual, economic, and administrative exploitation) of the patient and his companions.

- Commercial advertising of medical and pharmaceutical products by medical professionals, directly or indirectly (including the installation of promotional announcements in the workplace that has a commercial aspect or the presentation of promotional speeches for commercial products), is not allowed.

9.4 Fairness and impartiality

- Medical professionals should not engage in actions such as delaying appointments, providing faster services, and so on, in providing services to patients, with financial and nonfinancial incentives or for reasons such as financial affordability of some patients, because this is discrimination among patients.

- While observing fairness and justice among patients, it is necessary to pay special attention to people who are in vulnerable groups, including children, pregnant women, the elderly, mental patients, prisoners, mentally and physically disabled, and people without guardians.

- Medical professionals are obliged to provide health services to people suffering from certain diseases, including diseases that have a risk of transmission, in compliance with the rules and principles of safety like other patients. It is forbidden to dissuade patients from requesting health services in any way.

9.5 Honesty and integrity

- Medical professionals should try to maintain patients' trust in the profession and health professionals. In this context, it is necessary to provide the necessary information to the patients with complete honesty in all stages of diagnosis and treatment and avoid direct or indirect speech or behavior that involves deceiving the patients (even with the intention of benefiting the patient).

- Medical professionals, for the well-being of patients and their companions, should do their best to adjust the patient's time as accurately as possible during patient visits and respond to their needs as quickly as possible. In cases where patients have to wait to see the professionals providing health services for any reason, they should be provided with essential amenities (such as water, chairs to sit, and toilets) as much as possible.

- It is necessary for the medical professionals to give realistic hope and information to the patient, his family, and relatives while making a compassionate effort to alleviate the worries and fears of the patients and refrain from giving them false promises or hopes.

- Medical professionals are obliged to refrain from attracting patients with methods that require misleading advertisements, providing false or exaggerated information, or in any way that is against professional affairs.

9.6 Respecting the right to choose the recipients of health services

- It is necessary to respect patients' personal and religious beliefs in providing health services.

- All the information related to the patient that is necessary to know for the patient to make decisions about how to continue the diagnostic and treatment process and other life decisions should be provided to the patient or his substitute decision-makers based on the patient's level of literacy and condition, in a way that is understandable to the patient.

- In cases where the presentation of disease-related information includes bad news about the patient's health, it is necessary to give information to the patient using standard methods of "giving bad news". However, it is not justified to limit the patient's right to know all the information related to his health.

- It is necessary for medical professionals to guide patients to the best of their ability to obtain information about the criteria and foreseeable costs in the process of diagnosis and treatment.

- In addition to performing diagnostic and therapeutic interventions, it is necessary to provide necessary training in the field of how to continue the treatment, how to take the drugs, follow up the disease, the time of the next visits, the side effects of taking the drugs, the cases where the patient should go to the doctor or the emergency room of the hospital, lifestyle modification, and so forth. It should be provided to the patient.

- Medical professionals are obliged to respect the right of patients to freely and consciously choose the treatment method.The choice of patients in this field is limited to choosing among the options that are logical and correct from the scientific and technical point of view. However, respecting the patients' right to choose does not mean that the members of the organization must comply with every request of the patient; rather, it refers to the patient's right to choose from among the correct options available.

- Medical professionals are obliged to respect the patient's right to refuse the proposed treatments.The use of methods that require dishonest behavior to persuade the patient to accept treatment is prohibited.

- In cases where the patient does not accept life-sustaining treatments and may die or suffer serious injuries as a result of refusing treatment, the attending physician is obliged to use all his efforts to convince the patient. And finally, if the patient is not satisfied, he should inform the relevant authorities, including the hospital's ethics committee, about the matter. Critical emergency cases in which it is not possible to exchange information and obtain consent from the patient or his/her substitute decision-maker due to the urgency and risk of the patient's life are excluded from the inclusion of this issue.

- Medical professionals are obliged to prioritize saving the patient's life over other ethical rules, including the need to obtain informed consent, and provide services without wasting time in emergency cases where the patient's life is in danger. In emergency cases where the patient refuses to accept life-saving treatment despite the existence of a serious threat to his health and life, medical professionals are obliged to use their utmost efforts to convince the refusing patient to accept the treatment.

- To perform any medical intervention, if the person has reached the legal age and has the authority to make decisions, the informed consent of the person is sufficient and the consent of another person is not required. Cases of nontherapeutic medical intervention that has a serious and irreversible effect on a person's fertility or his marital relationship or with the possibility of a weak and long-term return, if the person is married, will be subject to the consent of the spouse. However, no medical treatment should be dependent on the consent of a person other than the patient or his/her substitute decision-maker.

9.7 Confidentiality and privacy

- Medical professionals are obliged to respect the patient's right to the confidentiality of all his information, including sensitive and nonsensitive information that is collected in any form, in different stages of diagnosis and treatment, or is provided to the treatment team in any way.

- Medical professionals are obliged to respect patients' privacy. Respecting patients' privacy requires refraining from all activities that patients consider to be a violation of their privacy. In this context, the members of the organization should refrain from actions such as examining the patient in the presence of other people, asking sensitive questions to the patients in the presence of others in a way that causes embarrassment to the patients, and unnecessary observation or touching of the patients, especially in the case of non-same-sex patients.

- Medical professionals are obliged to refrain from any investigation into the personal and family affairs of patients. It is necessary to avoid asking patients personal questions unrelated to the diagnosis and treatment of the disease. If it is necessary to ask questions that the patients may consider as an invasion of their privacy, for diagnosis and treatment, the necessity of the questions should be informed to the patients in simple and understandable language.

- Doctors are obliged to refrain from examining and visiting several patients at the same time in the examination room.

- Carrying out any kind of photography and filming of patients with the aim of preparing educational content, using in the research process (such as reporting specific cases) or treatment (such as photos taken for cosmetic surgery), preparing a movie, documentary, or news program and the like, is only allowed after obtaining permission from the patients.

In cases where the identity of the person is known, the obtained consent must be written.

The responsibility of any misuse of the video or images taken for the purpose of education or research is the responsibility of the medical and allied professionals who took the said video or photo.

- Information and samples related to the patient's body, such as radiographs, tissue samples, blood and biological fluids, and genetic content extracted from the body, are part of the patient's privacy, and their use is allowed for various purposes, such as medical and research purposes. Either the owner's consent has been taken, or the information and samples have been anonymized in a way that cannot be attributed to their owners.

9.8 Management of medical errors

- Medical professionals are obliged to use all their efforts to provide standard health services free from medical errors. In this context, it is necessary for all members to do their best to be aware of the common errors in their field of work and to prevent these errors as much as possible.

- Based on the right of patients to know information related to their health, medical professionals should accept the responsibility of their actions in case of an error that leads to damage and while apologizing and taking corrective and preventive measures, the origin of the error and the details related to it, including the causes and complications caused by the error to reveal to the patients.

- In order to maintain the mutual trust of the society and the medical profession, it is necessary for medical professionals, in cases of errors that lead to any kind of physical, psychological, social, and economic damage to patients, while avoiding any kind of concealment, with the agreement of the patient and voluntarily, for compensate for the damage caused by their mistake.

- Medical professionals are obliged to continuously monitor themselves in terms of physical and mental capabilities necessary to perform their professional duties correctly and completely. If for any reason, including fatigue, physical weakness, or mental weakness, the patient is likely to be harmed, they should refrain from performing the mentioned intervention as much as possible.

9.9 Communication with other colleagues

- Medical professionals are obliged to respect the rights of other colleagues and members of the medical team at all levels and to observe the utmost courtesy in their interactions with them.

- It is necessary for medical professionals to help their colleagues and other professionals providing health services as much as possible in order to solve the problems that arise in the field of professional behavior, clinical practice, and health.

- Medical professionals are obliged to teach their colleagues and other members of the health service team their knowledge and experience as much as possible. In cases where colleagues ask for advice from any member of the organization, it is necessary to give the answer of the professionals being consulted as soon as possible, in the best way and in such a way that the colleague seeking advice, upon receiving the advice answer, can clearly understand its content and use it in the course of providing the service.

- Medical professionals are obliged to refrain from any unconstructive criticism, mistakes, insults, and humiliation of other professionals, in any case and especially in the presence of patients and their companions.

- It is necessary for medical professionals to give priority to prevention over treatment in performing their professional duties and provide necessary preventive training to the recipients of health services.

9.10 Medical education and research

- It is necessary for medical professionals to make the improvement of human health along with respecting their dignity and rights as their main goal in research on human participants and prioritize the health and safety of the research participants during and after the research over all other interests.
- Medical professionals should only conduct human research in cases where they are confident that they have the necessary and relevant clinical expertise and skills for this work. The design and implementation of researches that are conducted on humans should be consistent with accepted scientific principles based on current knowledge and based on a complete review of available scientific resources and previous researches.
- If medical professionals who conduct human research realize during the research that the risks of participating in the research for the participants are greater than its potential benefits, the research must be stopped immediately.
- Medical professionals are required to obtain written informed consent from participants or their substitute decision-makers for research on humans.
- Medical professionals must make sure that the obtained consent is informed.
- For this purpose, they are obliged to inform the research participants of all the information that can be effective in their decision-making in an appropriate way.
- The informed consent form must be written for the participants in a simple and understandable language and contain the following information: "Research Title and Objectives," "Research Duration," "Research Method," "Funding Sources," "Any Possible Conflict of Interest," "Researcher's Organizational Affiliation," and "Profits and Losses that the Research is Expected to Include". Also, research participants should know that they can withdraw from the study at any time.
- Medical professionals must ensure that the consent obtained is free. Any behavior that includes threats, seduction, deception, or coercion for patients or other people in order to participate in the research is prohibited. Considering the need of the patients for their doctor, this issue should be considered more carefully about the patients being treated by the medical and allied professionals who intend to conduct therapeutic research on their patients.
- Medical professionals who are interested in research should do their best to respect the privacy and confidentiality of all the information of patients and participants in the research and prevent the unjustified dissemination of the information obtained and collected during the research.
- -Medical researchers are obliged to take all necessary measures to compensate for any possible damage to patients caused by participating in the research. In cases where the research is supported by pharmaceutical companies, it is necessary to ensure the full insurance coverage of the participants from the financial sponsor and then start the research.

- Medical research professionals are required to cover all the costs of actions that are purely research-related, from the research budget, and refrain from imposing any research costs on patients or using their health insurances.

10. Conclusion

In this chapter, the domains of professional behavior in medicine are briefly reviewed and important cases of these indicators are stated. Professional behavior in almost all general and specialized medical education capability frameworks exists, and most medical schools have included it in their curricula, but they still have challenges in teaching it. What emerges from the evidence is that model-oriented and rethinking are the most effective methods for teaching professional behavior. Educational methods will be effective when the educational environment (university and hospital) encourages professional behavior and prevents unprofessional behavior of people. It seems that a mentoring system is very necessary in the structure of general medical education to guide the formation of professional identity. By holding regular and continuous meetings with a fixed group of learners, the mentors provide feedback and guide their rethinking of their clinical experiences, and on the one hand, they help the learners adapt to the conditions of uncertainty, stress, and problems that occur to them and rehabilitate, and it helps to correct their behavior. In addition, mentoring helps to identify the challenges of the educational system that created the hidden curriculum. In a structure where students have short-term rotations in specialized and superspecialized departments, one cannot hope for effective training of professional behavior except with the mentoring system. Supportive environment and incentive policies, helping learners in resilience, and improving their personal growth are also other measures that can be effective in improving the professional behavior of learners.

Author details

Vida Seifouri
Razi University, Kermanshah, Iran

*Address all correspondence to: v.seifouri@razi.ac.ir; v.seifouri@gmail.com

References

[1] Kirk LM. Professionalism in medicine: Definitions and considerations for teaching. Proceedings (Baylor University Medical Center). 2007;**20**(1):13-16

[2] Saeedi Tehrani S, Nayeri F, Parsapoor A, Jafarian A, Labaf A, Mirzazadeh A, et al. Development of the first guideline for professional conduct in medical practice in Iran. Archives of Iranian Medicine. 2017;**20**(1):12-15

[3] Asghari F, Rahimi M, Nayeri FS, Samadi S, Alipour F, Labaf A, et al. Medical Professionalism: A Scenario-Based Guide. Tehran: Behdad; 2015

[4] Cruess RL. Teaching professionalism: Theory, principles, and practices. Clinical Orthopaedics and Related Research. 2006;**449**:177-185

[5] Schlesinger M. A loss of faith: The sources of reduced political legitimacy for the American medical profession. The Milbank Quarterly. 2002;**80**(2):185-235

[6] Kaczmarczyk JM, Chuang A, Dugoff L, Abbott JF, Cullimore AJ, Dalrymple J, et al. E-professionalism: A new frontier in medical education. Teaching and Learning in Medicine. 2013;**25**(2):165-170

[7] Bahaziq W, Crosby E. Physician professional behaviour affects outcomes: A framework for teaching professionalism during anesthesia residency. Canadian Journal of Anaesthesia. 2011;**58**(11):1039-1050

[8] Papadakis MA, Hodgson CS, Teherani A, Kohatsu ND. Unprofessional behavior in medical school is associated with subsequent disciplinary action by a state medical board. Academic Medicines. 2004;**79**(3):244-249

[9] Stark P, Roberts C, Newble D, Bax N. Discovering professionalism through guided reflection. Medical Teacher. 2006;**28**(1):25-31

[10] Cruess SR, Cruess RL. Professionalism must be taught. British Medical Journal (BMJ). 1997;**315**(7123):1674-1677

[11] Harden RM. Curriculum planning and development. In: Dent JA, Harden RM, editors. A Practical Guide for Medical Teachers. 4th ed. London, New York: Elsevier; 2013

[12] Hafferty FW, Gaufberg E. The hidden curriculum. In: Dent JA, Harden RM, editors. A Practical Guide for Medical Teachers. 4th ed. Edinburgh: Elsevier; 2013

[13] van Mook WN, van Luijk SJ, de Grave W, O'Sullivan H, Wass V, Schuwirth LW, et al. Teaching and learning professional behavior in practice. European Journal of Internal Medicine. 2009;**20**(5):105-111

[14] Sandars J. The use of reflection in medical education: AMEE Guide No. 44. Medical Teacher. 2009;**31**(8):685-695

[15] Menard L, Ratnapalan S. Teaching moment: Reflection in medicine: Models and application. Canadian Family Physician. 2013;**59**(1):105-107, 57-9

[16] Birden H, Glass N, Wilson I, Harrison M, Usherwood T, Nass D. Teaching professionalism in medical education: A Best Evidence Medical Education (BEME) systematic review. BEME Guide No. 25. Medical Teacher. 2013;**35**(7):1252-1266

[17] Passi V, Johnson S, Peile E, Wright S, Hafferty F, Johnson N. Doctor role modelling in medical education: BEME Guide No. 27. Medical Teacher. 2013;**35**(9):1422-1436

[18] Rademacher R, Simpson D, Marcdante K. Critical incidents as a technique for teaching professionalism. Medical Teacher. 2010;**32**(3):244-249

[19] Babasafari M, Marzooqi R, Faqih N, et al. Evaluating the professional ethics of Shiraz University professors from the perspective of graduate students and its medical sciences. Journal of Education and Ethics in Nursing. 2013;**2**(2):1-10

[20] Dehghani F, Salimi J, Zarezadeh Y, et al. Developing a curriculum pattern of professionalism for medical sciences students. Iranian Journal of Medical Education. 2020;**20**:484-499

[21] Valipour Khajehghyasi R, Sadeghimahalli F, Mohammadi M, et al. Evaluation of teaching professional ethics of professor from the viewpoint of medical and pharmacy students of Mazandaran University of Medical Sciences. JMED. 2021;**15**(4):224-233

[22] American Board of Internal Medicine. Project Professionalism. Philadelphia: ABIM; 1995

[23] Najafi H, Maleki H. An assessment of faculty Members' professional ethics from Students' viewpoint in Medical School of Shahed University. Journal of Medical Education Development. 2016;**9**(21):93-102

[24] Hamidvand A, Moazedi K, Enjoo SA. Ethical criteria in medical profession. Journal of Pizhūhish dar dīn va Salāmat. 2021;7(2):155-169. DOI: 10.22037/jrrh.v7i2.27213

Chapter 4

Professional Values and Ethics in Medical Education

Ebtihaj T. Nafea

Abstract

Medical ethics, professionalism and values have been commonly attached to medicine since its ancient era. These terms, although they differ, have been used in medical literature to refer to the right way to do the right thing by medical professionals. Professionalism was and still is one of the major aims of medical education. It refers to a complex process by which medical professionals acquire and apply the essential knowledge and skills together with acceptable values and ethics to serve society. However, teaching and assessing professionalism is not a straightforward mission. The complexity of it comes from its real nature being affected by many factors in multiple dimensions, including individual, interindividual and the larger societal or institutional levels. In this chapter, I describe the interaction between these factors after shedding light on the different interrelated terms. I also highlighted the advances and recommendations regarding teaching and assessment of professional values in the field of medicine.

Keywords: ethics, medicine, medical education, professionalism, values

1. Introduction

Ethical principles have long framed medicine. The Hippocratic Oath, 400 BC, reflected the constant goal of medicine '*I will use treatment to help the sick according to my ability and judgment; I will keep them from harm and injustice*'. This oath is based on beneficence, non-maleficence, justice and respect for the patient's autonomy with its two rules of confidentiality and veracity. Looking at this, medicine is commonly perceived as a respectable profession that best serves society. Doctors are expected to perform procedures and take decisions based on their professional education and training. They are usually assumed to do all that is right in the right manner. Therefore, certain values characterise medical professionals and even medical students as they collectively form a special society with specific characteristics. When we look at this society one would assume that they attain sophisticated knowledge and they have special skills that an ordinary individual would not easily acquire or apply. The white coats usually symbolise highly respected professionals. These professionals besides their knowledge and skills are commonly perceived as being wise and strive to do the right things. It is not uncommon for patients seeking treatment to trust their physicians and let them decide on and carry out the best options in the right manner based on their experience. The physicians' presented behaviour and ethical values are affected by multiple factors. Understanding the dynamic nature of professionalism would aid its teaching and assessment and therefore, its acquisition by medical professionals.

In this chapter, I describe ethics, morality and professionalism based on medical literature. In depth contemporary categorisation of medical values is discussed. I also highlighted the advances in teaching and assessing professional values.

2. What are the differences between ethics, morality and professionalism?

Ethics, morality and professionalism are frequently encountered terms when discussing what is right and wrong. Although sometimes these terms were used synonymously, there are some differences between them. I will describe these differences in a simple way. Members of a particular profession are governed by a set of values or principles, duties and obligations based upon standards of right and wrong. These sets of standards are known as *ethics*, and they are formulated by the governing council of a professional group. All professions have a known Code of Ethics that characterises professions and reflects a high level of trust between professionals and their clients [1]. *Morality* on the other hand reflects the individual values and conduct that people believe in when deciding good and bad behaviours. Morality is deeply rooted within the individuals themselves rather than being proposed by governing bodies [1]. The last term proposed here is *professionalism*. This term has a wider aspect when compared to ethics and morality. It includes both mastering biomedical aspects (knowledge and its proper application), psychometric aspects (mastering of specific skills) and humanistic aspects (attitude, behaviour, virtues and characteristics), desirable among professionals. The usual definition of a profession is that it is a vocational occupation characterised by specific knowledge and skills specially devoted to this specific field, which comprises autonomy and self-regulated bodies. All this knowledge and skills are serving the good of the public [2].

Medicine is a speciality which has long been known to focus on professionalism, representing a trustworthy relationship between physicians and their patients. Acceptable conduct or traits constituting professionalism were imperative to health professions. However, professionalism, per se, was not the focus of medical education 30 years ago. This state remained until the American Board of Internal Medicine (ABIM) started its humanism project in the early 1980s, which led to Project Professionalism in the mid-1990s [3]. Although professionalism is actually one of the 11 values encountered in healthcare professions literature [4], the term professionalism was also used synonymously in medical literature to refer to sets of values that are collectively acceptable by medical professionals. I suggest that using the term professionalism to refer to multiple professional values might reflect that medicine is an autonomous profession that is characterised by its ethics and values.

There is a large amount of literature on professionalism in medicine as old as 1890. However, these were mainly common advice to doctors and medical students towards doing what was socially acceptable and what was the right thing to do such as being honest and maintaining the patient's dignity as Cathell reported over a 100 years ago [5]. Professionalism was, and still is, generally perceived as a developmental value that medical students informally and passively catch from their educators [6]. Despite the increasing interest in professionalism, a consensus about the proper definition is still lacking in medical literature [3]. There are more than 20 different definitions for professionalism in medical literature reflecting the different aspects of it [3, 7].

Some of these definitions simply refer to the constitution of the contract between the profession and the society [8, 9]. Burak et al. [6] found 90 constituent elements of professionalism in their review of medical literature. Altruism, accountability, respect and integrity were among the most common elements. They identified three types of professionalism based on the nature of interaction. *Interpersonal professionalism* reflects meeting the demands for adequate contact with patients and other healthcare professionals. Elements such as altruism, respect, integrity, service, honour, honesty and compassion were related to this type. The other type is *the public professionalism*, which is expressed by meeting the demands society places on the medical profession. Elements related to this type include accountability, submission to an ethical code/moral commitment, excellence and self-regulation. The last type is *intrapersonal professionalism* perceived as meeting the demands to function in the medical profession as an individual including lifelong learning, maturity, morality, value of medical work intrinsically, humility and critique as common elements. The discipline that deals with the practical application of professional ethics is known as clinical medical ethics. Its main aim is always to ensure that the right and good decisions are taken for individual patients' cases, which in turn improve the quality of the healthcare provided [10].

3. What values are encountered in medical professions?

It is a common practice to refer to lists of values, traits and behaviours when discussing professionalism in medical education. This practice has its advantages and limitations. On one hand, analysis of the data having these lists of measurable behaviours that reflect certain values would formulate the basis for teaching and assessing medical professionalism for certification. However, there is a need to implement the internationally accepted and agreed-upon list of values to aid in teaching professionalism in medical curricula [11, 12]. On the other hand, it would be unwise to limit the definition of professionalism in such a manner. Focusing on these lists would mask the interactive and developmental process of professionalism.

Is attaining the listed behaviours enough to reflect the level of professionalism? To answer this question, we must immerse ourselves in professionalism and its sociological perspectives. Martimianakis [5] argued that there are competing and unstable factors affecting professionalism. These factors are related to the individual traits of the professional, the available facilities of the healthcare organisation and the power of assessing individuals related to race, gender and class.

As discussed earlier, a long time ago central values were attached to doctors such as beneficence, benevolence, respect and concern for patients, truthfulness, friendliness and justice when treating their patients [13]. Technical, interpersonal and humanistic values are all required to ensure the best care delivery to society [7]. To start discussing the professional values related to healthcare, we should highlight the definition of values. Values usually refer to the right and acceptable thing to do with a consensus in society. Values are prominent in everyday activities. They guide the evaluation of people, choices and actions and influence their behaviours [14].

The nature of the doctor-patient relationship was categorised by Drane [13] into 6 dimensions: *medical,* which represents diagnostic and therapeutic acts; *spiritual*, the verbal communication between the two; *volitional*, the decision of the doctor and the patient; *affective*, reflecting the feeling associated; *social*, the broader aspect of medicine towards the society; and lastly a *religious* role that sometimes played by doctors in some cases. We should also differentiate between personal values, which guide an individual's behaviour and personal choices [14], from professional values, which govern their behaviour as members of a profession [15]. Both types of values affect the decision-making process taken by clinicians. Therefore, personal and professional values are equally important to be clearly understood and assessed in medical education. Healthcare specialties share relatively similar professional values with some differences in prioritising them and focusing on specific profession-related ones. Common principles such as putting the patients' interests above self-interests, avoiding harm to patients and equitable access to healthcare, are shared and applied to all healthcare professions [16].

Understanding professional values is important to medical educators so that they can teach and ensure the development of these values in their students, which in turn guides them through their profession and highlights the importance of a patient-centred approach in healthcare [17]. Since 1985, Braithwaite and Law [18] identified ten broad values, or value types, which describe motivational goals responsible for the decision-making process in all cultures. Moyo et al. [4] proposed a theoretical framework of values applicable to health professions based on Schwartz's values model, which describes these values after adding an eleventh value type 'spirituality' to the list. However, this value type was not consistently perceived across cultures [19]. Moyo et al.'s Healthcare Practioner Values Framework aimed at implementing a universal and sharable framework through health professions, which can facilitate the delivery of integrated healthcare [4] and interprofessional practice [20]. This framework categorises certain values common in healthcare professions. **Figure 1** illustrates these healthcare practitioner values and their aligned values in the Schwartz model. The relations between these values were also described in the framework, adapted from the Schwartz model. Four motivational goals, each comprising a group of values, were described and their positions in the sphere reflect their relation. Adjacent goals show greater compatibility and their values related to each other, whereas, opposing goals in the sphere contain values with greater conflicting relations *e.g.* openness to change opposes conservation and self-enhancement opposes self-transcendence. The different values are categorised into four main groups of conflicting pairs as follows:

- Values that serve individual interests, which are known as *self-enhancement* conflict with values that serve collective interests referred to as *self-transcendence* values.

- Values that highlight independent thoughts and flexibility to change, which are known as *openness to change values* oppose values that emphasise self-restriction, order and resistance to change representing *conservation.*

Within these groups, there are 11 values derived from values presented by healthcare practitioners. These value types are namely: authority, capability, pleasure, intellectual stimulation, critical-thinking, equality, altruism, morality, professionalism, safety and spirituality [4].

In the proposed framework these values were structured as follows:

- Authority, capability and pleasure into the group of *self-enhancement values* as they emphasise advancing self-interests

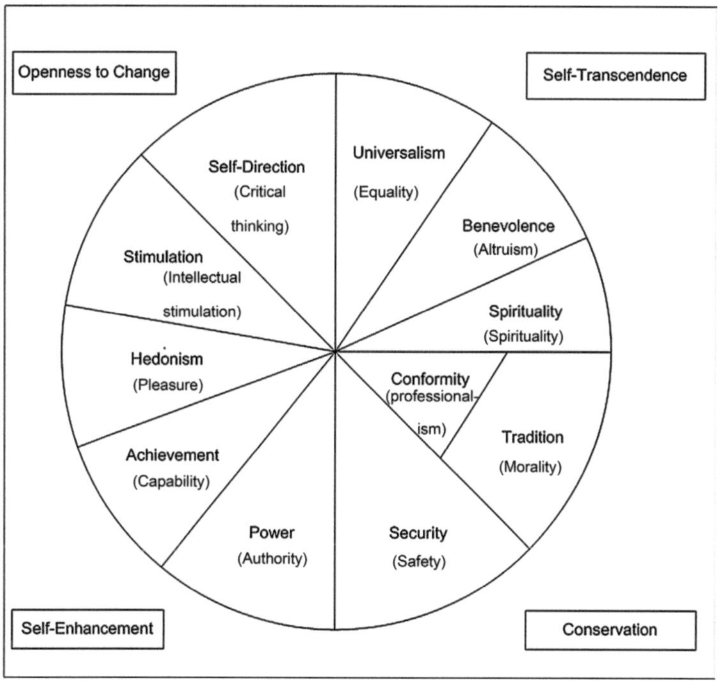

Figure 1.
The healthcare practitioner values framework. Adapted from Moyo et al. [4]. Motivational goals are present in frames at each quadrant of the sphere. Each goal comprises number of values. Values between brackets are special for the healthcare practitioner. They are written below their corresponding values commonly found in individuals derived from Schwartz's structure of value relations [19]. Adjacent values show greater compatibility. However, competing values are located opposite to each other. The projected behaviour of an individual is a result of the interaction between these values.

- Equality and altruism into *self-transcendence values* as they emphasise concern for the welfare and interests of others
- Critical-thinking, intellectual stimulation and pleasure are grouped into *openness-to-change values* as they emphasise independent action, thought
- New experiences; and spirituality, morality, professionalism and safety are grouped into *conservation values* as they emphasise order and preservation of traditions.
- Pleasure is placed in both *self-enhancement* and *openness-to change* groups, as it shares emphases with both groups

From the previous discussion of human values, we understand that the nature of the presented behaviour or action is based on the conflict or enhancement interaction between the different values. Therefore, applying clinical ethics is not a direct process. Rather, the interaction between many factors plays important roles in this process. Clinicians try to make their decisions based on medical and scientific facts. Moreover, the preferences, values and their nature discussed earlier, and the goals of both the physician and the patient are important. Their decision is also affected by external constraints, such as cost, limited resources and legal duties, that may shape or limit choices [10, 21].

4. Teaching medical ethics

Nowadays, the focus has been given to the humanistic values in medical literature and little to the technical ones, because the latter were kind of normally expected by patients when they seek medical treatments by healthcare services [22, 23]. With the changing goals of medicine towards a more patient-based approach, professional ethics should be applied besides clinical competency and dictate the physician-patient relationship [24]. As old as the 1970s medical educators reinforced the importance of teaching ethics. In the late 1980s and early 1990s, there were repeated calls for the formal education of medical ethics in medical schools [25]. Gazibara [26] described the need for a holistic approach in contemporary education. In this approach, certain important qualities were compared to the active components of human presence: the heart (values), head (knowledge) and hands (skills). All of these contribute to the values necessary for the development of professionalism.

Nevertheless, dilemmas and conflicting views are present as to whether ethics can be effectively taught or not. Can we anticipate that when medical ethics are taught, medical students will have ethical values when practising medicine? Is there a difference between good doctors and doctors who perform well? Is it a skill that can be taught and applied later in training or values that characterise the identity of medical professionals? These questions will lead us to think about the nature of ethical value education. The focus here would be the effect of individual values and personality. It was found that medical students caught for unprofessional behaviours during their undergraduate study were more inclined to do the same after they graduated [27]. This argument further stresses the effect of individual values that tend to be stable. Another issue surrounding the teaching of medical ethics is, if we can formally teach and assess ethics as tools present in the curriculum, are we neglecting socialisation in the development of these values? The complex and multidimensional nature of professionalism together with the present lack of consensus about what constitutes professionalism adds more difficulties to teaching it. In addition to all these factors, it would be unwise to underestimate the effect of hidden curriculum. A hidden curriculum can adversely affect the acquiring of ethical values in medical students when the teaching faculties do not appreciate the role of the hidden curriculum, which should be aligned with the formal instructions [25].

It is recommended that teaching medical ethics should start early in medical schools and continue throughout undergraduate and postgraduate study and training [1]. Instead of having lists of theoretical medical values, teaching ethical values should focus on applying them in clinical situations where they are practically applied in the real world [28]. Another recommendation in teaching medical ethics is giving full attention to hidden curriculum, by playing not only role models by the faculty but also by engaging all educators and students in making up a culture of medicine representing ethical values. Teaching ethical values is an integrative and comprehensive process. It should be directed towards raising sensitivity, providing knowledge, facilitating reflection, decision-making and improving action and behaviours [29]. This teaching still needs support from educational organisations. It could be facilitated by directing the learning towards relevant ethical problems regularly encountered in clinical settings and including modalities that encourage knowledge and skill development [30]. However, studies have indicated that there is low consensus among doctors in solving a wide range of ethical dilemmas encountered daily. This further indicates the need to address more ethical dilemmas, other than the classical dilemmas dealing with death and life, when teaching medical ethics [31].

There are different designs and course contents applied in medical schools regarding teaching medical ethics [30]. The different modalities involved, regular instructions and knowledge of the ethical values by lecturing and seminars, whether in person or online, the use of simulation and the presenting of real-life scenarios that involve students' discussions and reflection, with the latter proved to be more effective in developing the students' ethical behaviours [29, 30]. Problem-based learning and narrative reflections were also effective modalities that could be used to teach medical ethics [30, 32, 33]. Programs for teaching professional medical ethics have involved teams of faculty, residents and students in a longitudinal curriculum, focusing on the shared real experience of the members and the associated reflection by the students. This was thought to be effective in creating a medical school environment around professionalism [34]. Small group discussion is another modality that is thought to facilitate the discussion and reflection by students, especially for sensitive ethical issues that one would avoid discussing on a large scale [35]. Some innovative strategies, such as team-based learning were used to teach medical professionalism and found to be effective [36].

Searching the literature on medical education over the last five years led to some insights into how to develop ethical values in medical students. Some teaching experiences were found to enhance the appreciation of medical ethics by students, such as patient-led educational sessions. It also was found to aid the development of professional identity by role-playing [37]. Interventional workshops designed for fostering the development of professional values in medical students were also found to be effective in raising the students' positive attitudes, subjective norms, perceived behavioural control and intentions [38]. Measures to teach professional values may require adjustment of the medical curriculum to integrate more professional values of social accountability such as relevance, quality, equity and cost-effectiveness in the regular curriculum. These measures were found to be effective when they were applied to a problem based learning (PBL) curriculum [39]. In including the socialisation aspect of professionalism, I found a single study in medical education literature. This study used an innovative especially designed co-curriculum program with experiential learning opportunities in social settings during summer time. This was found to be effective in enhancing medical students' socialisation skills and teamwork, all of which contributed to their professional development and aided hominisation of medical curricula [40].

In conclusion, despite the serious attempts regarding the teaching of medical ethics, this practice is still not precise and not officially included in medical curricula [1]. Lastly, although one can assume that ethical education increases ethical sensitivity and the ability to detect an ethical problem, it is not obvious that education influences the development of ethical behaviour in medical students [41]. Therefore, the International Ottawa Conference Working Group on the Assessment of Professionalism recommended that research should be directed towards distinguishing what values are amenable and therefore can be taught from those which are deeply rooted in individuals and unable to amend. In this case, they should be included in the selection criteria during admission [42].

5. Assessing professionalism

As Arnold [3] stated '*Without solid assessment tools, questions about the efficacy of approaches to educating learners about professional behavior will not be effectively answered'*. Assessment of professional values is important to guide medical educators during the teaching of these values. It also helps to discover the level of professionalism in practitioners and facilitates the development of problem-solving skills [4]. Furthermore, research in the assessment of professionalism highlighted that high levels of professionalism were associated with better clinical performance by medical students [3, 4]. It is also highly recommended to implement formative assessment because medical students can benefit from the feedback that they receive during this process in managing their behaviours [42].

However, it is very difficult to agree upon the best practices to assess professionalism. The difficulty reflects the complex nature of this phenomenon. Professionalism encompasses a wide range of aspects, starting from the individual level, which includes attributes, capacities and behaviours. It extends to the interpersonal domain, involving interactions with other individuals and various contexts. Finally, it reaches the macro-societal level, where concepts like social responsibility, morality, political agendas and economic imperatives come into play. Additionally, these domains interact with each other. For instance, an individual's professional behaviour can be influenced by the context they are in, and similarly, the individuals within an institution can impact its collective professional values [42]. In order to assess this phenomenon, it would be beneficial to have lists of measurable behavioural expectations that are derived from each proposed value [43].

Regarding the available assessment tools for professionalism, a variety of them are developed and used for three specific intentions. Some of these tools were directed towards measuring professional behaviour as a component of clinical performance. The other type focuses on assessing professional behaviour, as a comprehensive entity in itself. The last type aimed to assess only single components of professionalism [3].

Professionalism was used to be assessed as a stable characteristic of an individual rather than assessing the professional behaviour of the individual [44]. Educators who support this view focus on assessing professionalism as a stable trait that is inherently present or sometimes developed in individuals. Therefore, they stress the importance of assessing professionalism for applicants in medical schools before their admission. For this group, who believe in the individualist approach, many tools are used, up to 88 scales and ratings [45]. Recent research showed that very short answer questions can also be used to assess ethical reasoning in medical students [36]. Most of the available assessment tools are criticised for their validity, reliability and their theoretical basis [46]. We now understand that professionalism is a complex construct that involves knowledge, values, attitudes and the ability to employ professional behaviours in real practice settings. Assessing professionalism as an individual construct by focusing on behaviour alone misses the complexity and multidimensional nature of it. In reality, the expressed behaviour resulted from conflicts between values, and for this specific reason, the assessment of professionalism should focus on the interaction and the conflicts between values and emotions that lead to specific professional or unprofessional behaviour, by medical students [47].

In contrast to the rigid assumption of individualist approach, a more fluid approach considers the interactions between individuals as an important factor responsible for the projected behaviours. In this view, professionalism is seen as an interpersonal process. Context is given more attention. Moreover, for the assessment tool to be reliable it also should consider the task-dependence nature of professionalism and its environmental factors [3]. Professionalism is perceived as being entirely created in interpersonal interactions. Assessment should take into account assessing students' cognitive problem-solving processes, monitoring learning environments as well as teacher-student relationships for interpersonal characteristics that could lead to unprofessional behaviours [45]. Therefore, educators who support this view argue that professionalism should not be assessed by scales at all [48]. This view suggests assessing professionalism by using data from multiple methods such as observation, conversations about behaviour and behavioural explanations, through narrative and text assessment besides using multi-source feedback [49].

The last view in the assessment of professionalism perceives it as a societal/institutional phenomenon. In this view assessment of professionalism should be directed towards fulfilling the expectations of the society or organisation. For that reason, values that constitute professionalism and their targeted assessment process may vary from one culture to another reflecting the different beliefs and interests [50]. In this view, professionalism should be assessed at a macro-level in terms of the function of groups, settings and institutions more than the micro-level of the individuals [5]. In 2011, the International Ottawa Conference Working Group on Professionalism concluded that assessing professionalism should be directed towards a multi-dimensional, multi-paradigmatic approach at different levels: individual, interpersonal and societal/institutional [42].

6. Conclusion

Medical professional values have been commonly discussed in medical literature. Medicine is well known for its ethics and values. However, we lack a consensus regarding the definition of professionalism and how it would ideally be taught and assessed. Listing medical professional values without deeply understanding their interaction and the multiple factors involved would mask the richness of professionalism phenomenon. Implementing the different perceptions of medical professionalism reflects its multidimensional nature and facilitates its teaching and assessment. In this chapter, I shed light on the contemporary view of medical values and the advances in teaching and assessing professionalism.

Conflict of interest

The authors declare no conflict of interest.

Author details

Ebtihaj T. Nafea
Taibah University, Madinah, Saudi Arabia

*Address all correspondence to: ebtihajnafea@gmail.com

References

[1] Desai MK, Kapadia JD. Medical professionalism and ethics. Journal of Pharmacology and Pharmacotherapeutics. 2022;**13**:113-118. DOI: 10.1177/0976500X221111448

[2] Evetts J. The concept of professionalism: Professional work, professional practice and learning. International Handbook of Research in Professional and Practice-Based Learning. 2014;**1**:29-56

[3] Arnold L. Assessing professional behavior: Yesterday, today, and tomorrow. Academic Medicine. 2002;**77**:502-515

[4] Moyo M, Goodyear-Smith FA, Weller J, Robb G, Shulruf B. Healthcare practitioners' personal and professional values. Advances in Health Sciences Education. 2016;**21**:257-286

[5] Martimianakis MA, Maniate JM, Hodges BD. Sociological interpretations of professionalism. Medical Education. 2009;**43**:829-837

[6] Burack JH, Irby DM, Carline JD, Root RK, Larson EB. Teaching compassion and respect: Attending physicians' responses to problematic behaviors. Journal of General Internal Medicine. 1999;**14**:49-55

[7] Wynia MK, Papadakis MA, Sullivan WM, Hafferty FW. More than a list of values and desired behaviors: A foundational understanding of medical professionalism. Academic Medicine. 2014;**89**:712-714

[8] Cohen JJ. Professionalism in medical education, an American perspective: From evidence to accountability. Medical Education. 2006;**40**:607-617

[9] Pavlica P, Barozzi L. Medical professionalism in the new Millenium: A physicians charter. La Radiologia Medica. 2003;**105**:263-265

[10] Siegler MA. Professional values in modern clinical practice. The Hastings Center Report. 2000;**30**:S19-S22

[11] Atienza MI. A comparison of four models of professionalism in medical education. The Asia Pacific Scholar. 2021;**6**:24

[12] Jegan R, Dierickx K. Ethics without borders: An analysis of national and international guidelines on ethics in basic medical education. Advances in Health Sciences Education. 2023;**28**:1-22

[13] Drane JF. Becoming a Good Doctor: The Place of Virtue and Character in Medical Ethics. Kansas City: Rowman & Littlefield; 1988. ISBN: 1556122098

[14] Rokeach M. The Nature of Human Values. Washington, DC: Free Press; 1973. ISBN: 0029267501

[15] Eddy DK, Elfrink V, Weis D, Schank MJ. Importance of professional nursing values: A National Study of baccalaureate programs. Journal of Nursing Education. 1994;**33**:257-262

[16] Beauchamp TL. The 'four principles' approach to health care ethics. Principles of Health Care Ethics. 2007;**29**:3-10

[17] Martin P, Yarbrough S, Alfred D. Professional values held by baccalaureate and associate degree nursing students. Journal of Nursing Scholarship. 2003;**35**:291-296

[18] Braithwaite VA, Law HG. Structure of human values: Testing the adequacy of the Rokeach value survey. Journal

of Personality and Social Psychology. 1985;**49**:250

[19] Schwartz SH. Universals in the content and structure of values: Theoretical advances and empirical tests in 20 countries. In: Advances in Experimental Social Psychology. Vol. 25. San Diego: Elsevier; 1992. pp. 1-65. ISBN: 0065-2601

[20] McNair RP. The case for educating health care students in professionalism as the Core content of Interprofessional education. Medical Education. 2005;**39**:456-464

[21] Nafea E. Clinical Reasoning in Dental Students: A Comparative Cross-Curricula Study. Nottingham, UK: The University of Nottingham; 2015

[22] Dossetor JB. Bioethics--Human values in health care: Trying to get it right. CMAJ. 1997;**157**:1689-1690

[23] Markakis KM, Beckman HB, Suchman AL, Frankel RM. The path of professionalism: Cultivating humanistic values and attitudes in residency training. Academic Medicine. 2000;**75**:141-149

[24] Pellegrino ED. The metamorphosis of medical ethics: A 30-year retrospective. JAMA. 1993;**269**:1158-1162

[25] Hafferty FW, Franks R. The hidden curriculum, ethics teaching, and the structure of medical education. Academic Medicine. 1994;**69**:861-871

[26] Gazibara S. "Head, heart and hands learning"-A challenge for contemporary education. The Journal of Education, Culture, and Society. 2013;**4**:71-82

[27] van Mook WNKA, Gorter SL, De Grave WS, van Luijk SJ, Wass V, Zwaveling JH, et al. Bad apples spoil the barrel: Addressing unprofessional behaviour. Medical Teacher. 2010;**32**:891-898

[28] Siegler M. A legacy of Osler: Teaching clinical ethics at the bedside. JAMA. 1978;**239**:951-956

[29] Lechasseur K, Hegg Mme S, Mbemba GIC, Caux C, Maltais C. Educational strategies supporting the development of ethical competence among nursing students: An Integrative Review. Quality Advancement in Nursing Education-Avancées en Formation Infirmière. 2023;**9**:4

[30] Andersson H, Svensson A, Frank C, Rantala A, Holmberg M, Bremer A. Ethics education to support ethical competence learning in healthcare: An integrative systematic review. BMC Medical Ethics. 2022;**23**:1-26

[31] Bringedal B, Rø KI, Magelssen M, Førde R, Aasland OG. Between professional values, social regulations and patient preferences: Medical doctors' perceptions of ethical dilemmas. Journal of Medical Ethics. 2018;**44**:239-243

[32] Pandya R, Shukla R, GoR AP, Ganguly B. Personal experience narratives by students: A teaching-learning tool in bioethics. Indian Journal of Medical Ethics [Internet]. 2016;**1**:144-147

[33] Buxton M, Phillippi JC, Collins MR. Simulation: A new approach to teaching ethics. Journal of Midwifery & Women's Health. 2015;**60**:70-74

[34] Lazarus CJ, Chauvin SW, Rodenhauser P, Whitlock R. The program for professional values and ethics in medical education. Teaching and Learning in Medicine. 2000;**12**:208-211

[35] Lee W, Choi S, Kim S, Min A. A case-centered approach to nursing ethics education: A qualitative study. International Journal of Environmental Research and Public Health. 2020;**17**:7748

[36] Guraya SS, Guraya SY, Doubell F-R, Mathew B, Clarke E, Ryan Á, et al. Understanding medical professionalism using express team-based learning; a qualitative case-based study. Medical Education Online. 2023;**28**:2235793

[37] Butani L, Sweeney C, Plant J. Effect of a patient-led educational session on pre-clerkship students' learning of professional values and on their professional development. Medical Education Online. 2020;**25**:1-6

[38] Guraya SS, Rashid-Doubell F, Fredericks S, Halabi MOO, Mallah SIY, Sefen JAN, et al. Changing professional behaviors in the digital world using the medical education E-professionalism (MEeP) framework—A mixed methods multicentre study. Frontiers in Medicine (Lausanne). 2022;**9**:1-14. DOI: 10.3389/fmed.2022.846971

[39] Dash NR, Taha MH, Shorbagi S, Abdalla ME. Evaluation of the integration of social accountability values into medical education using a problem-based learning curriculum. BMC Medical Education. 2022;**22**:1-7. DOI: 10.1186/s12909-022-03245-6

[40] Senok A, John-Baptiste A-M, Al Heialy S, Naidoo N, Otaki F, Davis D. Leveraging the added value of experiential Co-curricular programs to humanize medical education. The Journal of Experimental Education. 2022;**45**:172-190

[41] Cannaerts N, Gastmans C, de Casterlé BD. Contribution of ethics education to the ethical competence of nursing students: Educators' and students' perceptions. Nursing Ethics. 2014;**21**:861-878

[42] Hodges BD, Ginsburg S, Cruess R, Cruess S, Delport R, Hafferty F, et al. Assessment of professionalism: Recommendations from the Ottawa 2010 conference. Medical Teacher. 2011;**33**:354-363

[43] Lesser CS, Lucey CR, Egener B, Braddock CH, Linas SL, Levinson W. A behavioral and systems view of professionalism. JAMA. 2010;**304**:2732-2737

[44] Ginsburg S, Regehr G, Hatala R, McNaughton N, Frohna A, Hodges B, et al. Context, conflict, and resolution: A new conceptual framework for evaluating professionalism. Academic Medicine. 2000;**75**:S6-S11

[45] Lynch DC, Surdyk PM, Eiser AR. Assessing professionalism: A review of the literature. Medical Teacher. 2004;**26**:366-373. DOI: 10.1080/01421590410001696434

[46] Li H, Ding N, Zhang Y, Liu Y, Wen D. Assessing medical professionalism: A systematic review of instruments and their measurement properties. PLoS One. 2017;**12**:e0177321

[47] Gillam L, Delany C, Guillemin M, Warmington S. The role of emotions in health professional ethics teaching. Journal of Medical Ethics. 2013;**40**:331-335

[48] Ginsburg S, Regehr G, Mylopoulos M. From Behaviours to attributions: Further concerns regarding the evaluation of professionalism. Medical Education. 2009;**43**:414-425

[49] Rees CE, Knight L. V the trouble with assessing students' professionalism: Theoretical insights from Sociocognitive psychology. Academic Medicine. 2007;**82**:46-50

[50] Ho M-J, Yu K-H, Hirsh D, Huang T-S, Yang P-C. Does one size fit all? Building a framework for medical professionalism. Academic Medicine. 2011;**86**:1407-1414

Section 3

Contemporary Teaching Methods

Chapter 5

Immersive Explorations: Transformative Experiences in Inter-Professional Education through Scenario-Based Learning

Aysel Başer, Ömer Faruk Sönmez and Hatice Şahin

Abstract

This chapter discusses the importance of scenario-based learning in interprofessional education and its transformative effects from theory to practice. The literature review shows that there is a growing interest and importance in this field between 2006 and 2023. Scenario-based learning offers students and health professionals the opportunity to develop practical skills through real-world scenarios. Educational theories (behaviorism, cognitivism, constructivism, connectionism, and experiential learning) support the design and implementation of this learning approach. Key principles of scenario writing include setting learning objectives, relevance to the target audience, realism, participant-centered development, inclusion of complex cognitive skills, use of activities and tools, detailed and clear descriptions, encouragement of reflective and critical thinking, evaluation, and feedback mechanisms. Ideal interprofessional education scenarios should be based on interprofessional knowledge exchange, be realistic, and develop students' problem-solving and decision-making skills. This process should be standardized through scenario templates and continuously reviewed. In this section, where all the theoretical knowledge is put into practice, an example of a workshop and an example of a scenario prepared in the workshop are presented.

Keywords: health education, interprofessional education (IPE), scenario-based learning (SBL), scenario writing principles, workshop example, medical education

1. Introduction

Interprofessional education is a learning model that emphasizes the sharing of knowledge and skills between two or more different professional groups. In the ever-changing environment of healthcare, Interprofessional Education (IPE) is becoming increasingly important. This chapter focuses on the intricacies of IPE scenario writing for new graduates in preparation for the complexities of collaborative practice in healthcare settings. We begin by examining the basic principles of IPE and highlighting the importance of promoting a collaborative, patient-centered approach among health professionals.

At the center of the discussion is the art and science of scriptwriting, combining theoretical knowledge with practical application. This chapter aims to guide educators in creating realistic, engaging, and educational scenarios that will effectively prepare undergraduate students for the challenges of interprofessional teamwork. Through these scenarios, students can experience the dynamics of healthcare settings and gain valuable insight into the communication, coordination, and ethical issues necessary for quality patient care.

In this journey of discovery, we highlight the impact of well-crafted scenarios on student engagement, critical thinking, and the development of a collaborative generation. Our aim is not only to inform but also to prepare tools to create effective learning experiences that inspire the next generation of healthcare professionals.

In this section, interprofessional education is emphasized as a key component and the role of scenario-based learning in this context and how the sample scenarios were developed are discussed in detail. Within the scope of experience sharing, the importance of scenario-based learning, scenario writing processes, and sample scenario development experiences were shared in detail.

2. Interprofessional education: definition and importance

Interprofessional education is a learning process in which professionals from different professions such as health, social engineering, communication, etc. come together to learn and teach through each other, sharing experience and knowledge. This type of education is critical for solving complex problems and promoting effective communication [1, 2]. By its very nature, interprofessional education is an educational strategy in which different health professionals benefit from their own knowledge, skills, and attitudes as well as the knowledge, skills, and attitudes of other health professionals with whom they receive training and, most importantly, from their professional and educational experiences. When this interaction is created, the existing knowledge, skills, and attitudes of individuals change radically, enabling them to gain new gains through this interaction and reflection [3, 4]. IPE provides opportunities for students and professionals to understand the roles, responsibilities, and perspectives of different disciplines and to adopt a patient-centered approach. In the literature, there are many learning methods for the implementation of interprofessional education. One of the key aspects to improving students' interprofessional collaboration, communication, and understanding of professional roles, values, ethics, and team-based patient care is to integrate interactive elements into teaching and learning. These methods include educational approaches such as scenario-based learning, peer learning, team-based learning, team-based case analysis, small group activities, problem-based learning, role-playing, digital learning platforms, videos, and simulation. The vast majority of these methods are actually based on scenario and team learning in IPE [5–8].

Student-centered, active learning strategies such as team-based learning, scenario-based learning, and problem-based learning are reported to be increasingly used in health professions classrooms [7, 9]. It was stated that in order to achieve maximum efficiency with these approaches, people should have knowledge about the theoretical background of the subject before the lesson, and the time allocated in these programs should be organized in a way to support collaborative learning [9, 10]. Especially in educational activities involving students from different disciplines, it is stated in the literature that students should interact with each other in small groups and teams while discussing or working, and as a result of this interaction, feedback should be given about the product produced by the teams [7, 11]. Although the level of evidence is low, the positive change in student attitudes supports the continued inclusion of IPE in health professional education to improve collaboration skills and patient care outcomes [12].

The most commonly used scenario-based learning (SBL) program in interprofessional education helps students develop their ability to analyze situations and generate solutions [13]. It is an educational approach that utilizes real-life scenarios. This method involves students working together to analyze and solve problems based on realistic situations and allows them to apply their knowledge and skills in a practical context. SBL has been recognized as an effective strategy to promote deeper learning and understanding as it provides students with the opportunity for active learning and critical thinking [14].

The role of scenario writing in interprofessional education is to shape a future that improves some aspects of the present. Scenario writers formulate their ideas by visualizing them within an interprofessional reality. These scenarios describe not only what reality could be like, but also improvements in interprofessional education and how they could be realized. Creative scenarios are one of our most effective tools, like knowledge, to accelerate and strengthen interprofessional relationships; they are important for repairing relationships that break down faster than is usually recognized [15].

3. Scenario-based learning: basic principles

A scenario provides a systematic and narrative description of a particular future. In education, scenarios can provide realistic and feasible alternative futures, enabling health professionals to think and learn in complex decision-making processes. This helps participants to assess situations from different perspectives, consider possible outcomes, and develop strategic thinking skills under uncertainty. For example, a scenario could examine the possible outcomes of different treatment approaches in the event of a specific health crisis, so that professionals can make the most appropriate decision among various scenarios [16].

Scenario-based learning is an effective teaching strategy that provides students with learning opportunities around a specific scenario or story This method allows students to better understand and apply knowledge by using real-world scenarios [14, 17].

Scenario-based learning is emerging as an effective tool in global health education. SBL uses scenarios that mimic real-world conditions, assigning participants a specific role and engaging them in a series of problem-solving or situation exploration activities around a realistic story. This approach helps learners develop their cognitive, metacognitive, and affective skills [14].

Nowadays, the use of scenarios in healthcare education has become an indispensable learning tool for students. As communication errors and misunderstandings pose a critical challenge to improving healthcare delivery, scenario writing in interprofessional education is becoming increasingly important to overcome these challenges [15, 18].

In the context of interprofessional learning, the act of scriptwriting requires creativity, and a multiprofessional approach should be adopted. Creativity is defined in the literature as a phenomenon that includes at least four basic characteristics. First, it produces something original, that is, it is different and innovative. It is also useful for improving an existing situation and is valuable because of the improvement it brings. Creativity is a multifaceted phenomenon that results in some kind of tangible or intangible product. It is a process in which each individual's creativity needs to be assessed and utilized because scriptwriting is a creative activity that is fed by different perspectives. Creative thinking involves a range of cognitive abilities that interact with each other. These abilities include generating a variety of ideas quickly, shifting to different concepts with mental flexibility, generating statistically rare and unique responses, conducting detailed analyses, and keeping an open mind. These cognitive capacities are thought to work integratively through collaboration. These capacities are developed in a collaborative effort through the interaction of people from different areas of expertise and approaches to problem-solving. As shown in the following section, the integration of these attributes, each of which is critical to the development of a creative scenario, is important for effectively guiding the creative process [15].

The aim of this study is to emphasize how scenario writing is critical to enhance communication, increase understanding, and improve educational processes among health professionals and to provide an interprofessional perspective to understand the impact of scenarios used in interprofessional education on student diversity and the health system.

4. Sharing experience on scenario development in interprofessional education

The theoretical background of the scenarios and the planned workshop was tried to be created with the literature on scenario writing in interprofessional education, and a workshop booklet was prepared with the information in the literature and designed to be used as a guide in the trainer meetings. The discussions were carried out with the concept framework prepared with the support of the literature, areas of competence in IPE, scenario-based training examples, and measurement and evaluation tools in the literature were compiled and shared with the faculty members at the workshop.

4.1 Findings from the literature review

As a result of the review of studies on scenario writing in interprofessional education and the Google school literature search in the field of scenario-based interprofessional education, a total of 39 articles were accessed between 2006 and 2023. Of these 39 articles, 9 are related to simulation applications but do not provide direct information about the use of scenarios. Most of the remaining 30 articles were published in 2023 (n:12; 40%) and 2022 (n:4; 13.33%), and the articles published in these years constitute more than 50% of the total. When all 30 articles are read, it is seen that 26 of them use scenarios in simulation applications, but no detailed information about scenario-based applications is given. When four articles were analyzed, the information in the **Table 1** below was obtained [8, 17, 19, 20].

Çelik et al. has implemented a scenerio based peer-learning approach in their study with European dental studentsi, which has been significantly motivating and echanching the readiness of the cohort [21].

These findings indicate that the scenario-based learning approach is gaining increasing attention and importance in interprofessional education. The articles focus on innovative training methodologies that allow learners to develop practical skills

DOI: http://dx.doi.org/10.5772/intechopen.114295

Article names	Authors	Published in Journal	Year of Publication	Objective	Conclusion	Scenario used	Professions and students mentioned in the article	Methods used	Practical applications
Encouraging Study in Health Sciences: Informing School Students Through Interprofessional Healthcare Simulations [19]	Christian Moro, Charlotte Phelps	Simulation in Healthcare	31/05/2023	The article does not mention specific interprofessional training scenarios.	Case-based learning with inter-professional hands-on experiences is effective in introducing students to future work options and career pathways in primary and allied health.	Participants worked on 3 simulated scenarios during the 1-day event.	"Health Simulation Experience" introduces high school students to careers in healthcare.	Using a case-based learning approach	The "Health Simulation Experience" is an effective way to inform high school students about careers in health. The use of case-based learning with inter-professional hands-on experiences is an effective approach to introduce students to future work options and career paths in primary and allied health care.
Engaging Student Learners in Interprofessional Simulations using Halloween-	Chase DuBois	Interprofessional Practice & Education	19/07/2023	The article describes the development and implementation of Halloween-themed interprofessional	The largest perceived change was observed in Communication.	Scenarios addressed cardiac arrest and CPR/AED skills, opioid overdose and Narcan	Health students from various disciplines such as athletic training, biology, clinical research, exercise science,	Single group post-test questionnaire design.	Improving communication skills in health students

Article names	Authors	Published in Journal	Year of Publication	Objective	Conclusion	Scenario used	Professions and students mentioned in the article	Methods used	Practical applications
Themed Scenarios [20]				simulation scenarios for healthcare students to develop their emergency management and teamwork skills.		treatment, emphasizing bleeding control and identifying hazards in the home environment for patient safety.	wellness, medicine, nursing, public health, recreational therapy, respiratory therapy and social work participated in the simulations.		
Patient safety interprofessional education program using medical error scenarios for undergraduate nursing and medical students in Korea [8]	Hea Kung Hur Ki Kyong Kim, Young Mi Lim, Junghee Kim, Kyung Hye Park, Yon Chul Park	Journal of Interprofessional Care	08/03/2023	The article discusses a patient safety interprofessional education program that uses medical error scenarios to enhance patient safety motivation and interprofessional learning attitudes among medical and nursing students.	The results of the medical scenario review of the patient safety IPE program showed increased motivation for patient safety among students and contributed to improving IPE learning attitudes by enhancing teamwork and collaboration.	The patient safety IPE program uses medical error scenarios.	The study aimed to improve attitudes to interprofessional learning among medical and nursing students.	Lectures, case studies, role-play and simulation activities	Improved motivation for patient safety among students
Does Interprofessional Scenario-Based	Marit Hegg Reime, Morten	Journal of Multidisciplinary Healthcare	22/12/2022	To investigate readiness for interprofessional	Our sample of Norwegian healthcare	Hypovolemic shock, anaphylactic	The study included undergraduate	A pre-test-post-test	One-day scenario-based simulation

DOI: http://dx.doi.org/10.5772/intechopen.114295

Article names	Authors	Published in Journal	Year of Publication	Objective	Conclusion	Scenario used	Professions and students mentioned in the article	Methods used	Practical applications
Simulation Training Change Attitudes Toward Interprofessional Learning – A Pretest-Posttest Study [17]	Aarflot, Fred-Ivan Kvam			learning (IPL) among Norwegian healthcare students at undergraduate, graduate, and postgraduate levels before and after participating in a one-day scenario-based simulation training course.	students shows readiness for IPL. The RIPLS has the ability to measure important changes in attitudes both within each profession and across professions.	reaction, a child with a febrile seizure and low blood sugar, and a trauma patient who lost consciousness due to increased intracranial pressure	and graduate nursing students as well as medical students who participated in a one-day scenario-based simulation training course.	survey design was used.	training was used as an intervention method. The practical applications of this training aimed to improve patient observation, clinical reasoning, problem-solving, leadership, teamwork, communication, prioritization, delegation, and medication administration skills, with participants experiencing both participant and observer roles.

Table 1.
Findings from the literature review.

through real-world scenarios. By focusing on scenario-based interprofessional education, the articles emphasize the importance of educational design and facilitation. This approach can help students and experienced healthcare professionals develop teamwork skills and support the effective use of simulation technologies. In summary, these articles show that scenario-based interprofessional education plays a critical role in health professional education and how simulation can transform this field [8, 17, 19, 20].

The use of scenarios in interprofessional education is considered a teaching strategy. When designing teaching strategies, the adult learning theory, which is considered within the constructivist theory [22], active learning theory [23], and experience-based learning theories [24] are also utilized [25]. Other educational theories underpinning SBL design and implementation include [14]:

Behaviorism: Emphasizes learning through repetitive practice and measures the learner's performance against specified learning objectives. This approach is useful in teaching cognitive skills for tasks that require automatization.

Cognitivism and Constructivism (constructivism, cognitivism): In these approaches, where knowledge is treated as an individual construct, learners are expected to actively process information and relate it to their existing knowledge in order to make sense of new information. SBL enables learners to explore knowledge interactively.

Connectivism: Proposes that learning is a process that occurs by making connections between information sources (nodes). SBL supports this theory by enabling learners to make connections between different sources and forms of knowledge.

Experiential learning: It focuses on the active participation of the learner and learning through an action-reflection cycle. SBL reinforces this approach by offering learners the opportunity to practice and receive feedback in a safe environment.

SBL design and implementation, based on educational theories, helps to understand the learning process and realize effective practices. This approach can be applied to global health-related topics, especially in complex and risky environments, for example in areas such as disaster medicine and humanitarian health. Moreover, SBL offers a cost-effective solution to increase equitable access to global health education by reducing training costs in the long term compared to traditional methods. Therefore, SBL is seen as an important tool in achieving global health goals [14].

Based on these theories, the following are the basic principles obtained during scenario writing as a result of the literature review.

5. Basic principles of scenario writing in interprofessional education

The basic principles of scenario writing in interprofessional education identified after the literature review are given below [5, 6, 8, 14, 17, 19, 20, 26–29].

Identifying learning objectives: The scenario should be in line with the identified learning objectives. Scenarios need to be developed in such a way that they address interprofessional rather than vocational learning objectives. However, they should not prevent other learning points from emerging. The learning objectives should be appropriate to the participants' needs and interprofessional competencies. They can cover a variety of areas such as human factors and medical or clinical issues.

Diversity and appropriateness of the target audience: Interprofessional scenarios should target participants from different professional groups and be appropriate to their needs and knowledge levels. It is important that the scenario is appropriate to the needs of the target group in terms of interprofessional competencies rather than their professional knowledge and skill level.

Realism: The scenario should be constructed to reflect real-life situations, organized, and implemented in a realistic way. The realism of the scenarios is important to enhance the participants' experience and enable them to easily adapt them to their clinical practice. It is important to have scenarios that require interprofessional collaboration. These scenarios may include dramatic moments or conflictual situations that will elicit emotional responses from learners. The scenario should be designed to keep learners constantly engaged and enrich the learning experience.

Participant-centered scenario development: Scenarios should be structured to include communicating with patients, family members, caregivers, and health professionals in a sensitive and responsible manner (interprofessional communication practice); using one's knowledge of one's own role and the roles of other health professionals to assess patients' needs (roles and responsibilities); applying principles of team dynamics to perform effectively in different team roles (teamwork); and practicing with professionals from other disciplines while maintaining mutual respect and shared values (interprofessional practice values). The scenario should include the perspectives and collaboration of different disciplines and professions.

Embody complex mental skills: These should include skills such as problem-solving, critical thinking, synthesis, and evaluation. By providing limited information to scenario participants, scenarios should be written that allow them to examine the situation and gather more information on their own.

Using activities and tools: Activities such as discussion, role play, and simulation should be utilized.

Detailed and clear descriptions: Characters, places, and events in the script should be described clearly and in detail.

Promote reflective and critical thinking: Participants should reflect on their personal, social, and professional values.

Evaluation and feedback: The scenario should have mechanisms for evaluation and feedback. In an effective SBL, feedback is one of the most critical elements of the learning process, enabling learners to receive explanatory feedback on their actions. Explanatory feedback enhances learning more than correct or incorrect feedback and can increase learner engagement. It is important that the scenarios include elements to assess the competence areas identified for interprofessional education (collaboration, teamwork, ethics communication skills, etc.).

Scenarios should be written on a detailed and reusable template.

5.1 Ideal interprofessional education scenario

Interprofessional education (ITA) scenarios should be based on learners' knowledge levels and interprofessional knowledge exchange. They should be designed to be appropriate to the level of knowledge of learners from each professional group, with sufficient theoretical background and a structure that can be associated with prior knowledge. In order to facilitate the achievement of the intended learning objectives, frequently encountered situations in society should be selected as case studies and their biological, psychological, and social aspects should be discussed with a multidisciplinary approach. The scenario should include detailed time, place, and identity information to increase realism; it should be supported with visual materials; and a language appropriate to social ethics should be used. The flow should follow the natural sequence of clinical practice. Analytical reasoning skills should be encouraged for simple problems and intuitive reasoning skills for complex situations. IPE mentors should develop scenarios with detailed and guided notes, including guiding questions to ensure that students achieve their learning objectives. These scenarios, with careful attention to spelling and grammar, should serve as ideal learning materials that develop students' problem-solving and decision-making skills and prepare them for real-life and professional practice. This process should be standardized with a scenario template and continuously reviewed by the team or committee [5, 6, 8, 26–29].

To summarize; when developing an interprofessional education scenario;

Scenarios should be prepared according to learning outcomes and competence areas identified in interprofessional education.

Not every scenario has to cover all competencies.

Scenarios should be written in accordance with real patient histories and students' cultures.

Scenarios may contain dramatic moments or conflicting situations that will cause students to react emotionally, but they should be written by establishing cause-effect relationships that do not allow for discussion.

Scenarios should focus on specific team-based issues. Examples of dysfunctional or poor teamwork, especially negative events resulting from communication breakdowns and lack of cooperation, can be good triggers for discussion and learning.

6. Scenario development in interprofessional education

The scenario should be developed jointly by the representatives of the faculties and departments where it is planned to be used. First of all, a workshop or meeting should be organized with the participation of at least one trainer representing all departments that will take part in interprofessional education.

6.1 Pre-workshop preparation

The purpose, title, and teaching method of our training program were determined through qualitative interviews conducted during the needs analysis phase. As a result of the literature review after the title selection, it was decided to address especially medical error scenarios and situations where medical errors may occur in interprofessional education (IPE) in accordance with the World Health Organization's 2010 recommendation that patient safety should be included in educational curricula to prevent medical errors. The main aim of the program is to enable students to gain knowledge, skills, and attitudes about interprofessional patient safety. Prior to the scenario development phase, the workshop design, scenarios, and evaluation methods were prepared, supported by literature research by five medical educators. The information obtained as a result of these preparations was collected in a booklet. To facilitate educators' contribution to the workshop, a trainer's guide was created, providing information on interprofessional education, core competencies, local and global examples, scenario-based learning, and assessment tools. The clinical scenarios in this guide aim to help health professionals better understand each other's roles and responsibilities and recognize the importance of teamwork and collaboration. The scenarios reinforce the concept and theories of Interprofessional Education (IPE) by putting them into practice. These scenarios can be used for small group activities and simulations in both undergraduate education and continuing professional development. Scenario-based education (SBE) is seen as an effective method for health professional students to acquire the competencies they will need in their careers, offering students the opportunity to work together and achieve common goals. Moreover, this method provides students with valuable experiences by providing a broad perspective on the roles and responsibilities of different professions in healthcare [30, 31]. In light of this information, scenario-based learning is an important tool to enable health professionals to learn interactively and to strengthen interprofessional collaboration.

Scenario development in interprofessional education workshop example (**Table 2**).

Session 1: Introduction, Discussion, and Meeting Expectations
Duration 15 min
Description: Meeting of educators from the Faculty of Medicine, Dentistry, Health Sciences
Objectives: Introducing the participants to each other and collecting expectations **Activities:** Short introductions of the participants. Receiving expectations with the help of software
Session 2: Deciding on Context and Conceptual Framework
Duration 60 min
Description: Introducing the concept of interprofessional education and establishing the conceptual framework
Objectives: To give information about the importance and aims of interprofessional education. To introduce the role of script writing in interprofessional education. **Activities:** An interactive presentation about interprofessional education and screenwriting. Group discussion on the characteristics of good screenwriting.
Session 3: Identifying the Competencies of the Interprofessional Education Program
Duration 30 min • Individual study (15 min) • Identification of competence areas with common consensus (15 min)
Description: Determination of program competencies in accordance with national and international core competencies
Objectives: To identify and agree upon a set of core competencies essential for effective interprofessional education (IPE) in healthcare. To understand how these competencies can be integrated into educational scenarios to promote collaborative practice among health professionals. To design educational activities that foster the development of identified IPE competencies. **Activities:** Introduction to IPE competencies: It starts with a presentation that outlines what IPE competencies are, why they are important, and how they contribute to the quality of healthcare delivery. Group discussion and brainstorming: It encouraged participants to consider IPE competencies that address gaps or challenges in current healthcare practice. Competency mapping exercise: Participants are tasked with mapping out how the competencies they have identified can be integrated into educational scenarios. This includes detailing specific learning objectives that align with each competency, and proposing methods for teaching and assessing these competencies. Competency prioritization and selection: Participants present their proposed competencies and the rationale behind their selection to the entire workshop. It was used techniques like voting or consensus-building exercises to finalize the list of competencies.
Session 4: Creation of patient scenarios suitable for planned core competence and qualifications
Duration: 60 min. • Presentation (20 min.) • Working on scenarios (40 min.)

Description: To make suggestions for scenario writing to be used in interprofessional education and to develop scenarios to be used in education
Objectives: Participants to develop their own scenarios. Creating scenarios that emphasize interprofessional cooperation and communication. **Activities:** Participants develop the drafts created by the program managers. Each participant shares his/her scenario with other participants and receives feedback. Evaluation of the scenarios in terms of realism, educational value, and interprofessional integration.
Session 5: Designing Assessment Tools for Scenarios
Duration: 60 min. • Sharing the prepared sample scenario and introduction to educational assessment methods (20 min) • Working on the Measurement Evaluation Tool (40 min)
Description: Sharing of sample scenarios and measurement evaluation tools prepared by program managers and development of materials prepared as a group
Objectives: To design assessment tools that measure the achievement of learning objectives in developed scenarios. To inform participants about effective assessment methods and teach them how to integrate these methods into their scenarios. To evaluate the alignment of scenarios with real-world healthcare practices. **Activities:** Introduction to educational assessment methods: A brief presentation introducing effective measurement and assessment methods. Examples might include multiple-choice questions, true/false questions, short answer questions, self-assessment surveys, 360-degree feedback, portfolio assessments, and performance assessments under observation. Scenario-based assessment design: Participants work self to design unique assessment tools for their developed scenarios. Each participant creates assessment tools that align with the learning objectives of their scenario. Participants discuss how their scenario's learning objectives align with their measurement and assessment tools and develop a plan. Development and application of assessment tools: Each participant shares their designed assessment tools with other participants, helping to create a collection of scenario-based assessment tools. Review and finalization of assessment tools: Participants revise their assessment tools considering the feedback received and create their final versions.
Session 6: Evaluation and closing
Duration: 15 min.
Description: Collect feedback from the participants to make an overall evaluation of the workshop.
Objectives: To make an overall evaluation of the workshop. To collect feedback from the participants. Activities: Participants give verbal feedback on all sessions of the workshop.

Table 2.
Scenario development workshop on interprofessional education.

6.1.1 Workshop objective

The goal is to ensure that participants who serve as educators in undergraduate and postgraduate education across all fields at higher education institutions train health professionals (such as Dentistry, Medicine, Health Sciences, Nursing, Physical Therapy and Rehabilitation, Nutrition, and Dietetics, etc.) become acquainted with the concept of interprofessional education, gain knowledge about the processes related to integrating it into their own educational programs, and acquire the skill of writing scenarios to be used in interprofessional education.

6.1.1.1 Session 1: Introduction, discussion, and meeting expectations

Ten faculty members actively serving in educational roles at the Faculty of Medicine, Dentistry, and Health Sciences (Departments of Nutrition and Dietetics, Physiotherapy, and Nursing) were invited, and seven faculty members accepted the invitation and participated in the workshop.

6.1.1.2 Session 2: Decision-making and conceptual framework development

6.1.1.2.1 Presentation

What is interprofessional education, its aims, and objectives? (10 mins).

Providing information on national and international core competency areas (10 mins).

In the literature, national core education and international interprofessional education framework programs have been evaluated. Among these framework programs, the framework presented by CAIPE is identified as the most commonly used framework for interprofessional competencies [4] and the introduction of other framework programs has been conducted [2, 32–40].

Information about professional roles and responsibilities (10 mins).

Deciding on the purpose, outcomes, and the faculties and departments that will be covered by this education program (20 mins).

An interactive presentation about screenwriting (10 mins).

6.1.1.3 Session 3: Identifying the competencies of the interprofessional education program

Individual work to identify program competencies and qualifications in accordance with the national and international core competency areas mentioned in the previous session (15 mins).

Determining faculty core competency areas with the collective contribution of all educators: reaching a consensus to establish a single set of core competencies and qualifications (15 mins).

6.1.1.3.1 Determined program core competencies for Turkey

Professional roles and responsibilities: It is essential for an individual to understand their own role and the roles and responsibilities of other health personnel related to their profession. For the effective delivery of health services and the advancement of public health, it is important for individuals to know their own duties and those of other health professionals, as well as how professional roles complement each other. This understanding ensures the harmony of roles and responsibilities, which is a common competency across most health professions [38].

Interprofessional ethics and values: This involves collaborating with individuals from different professional groups to ensure mutual respect and the preservation of common values. Those working in the health sector must learn to share and uphold mutual respect and common values to work effectively with others. This includes recognizing personal or colleague-originated biases and misconceptions and valuing the opinions and suggestions of other health professionals as much as one's own [38].

Interprofessional team and teamwork: To plan, deliver, and evaluate patient/community-centered care and public health programs and policies that are safe, timely, efficient, effective, and equitable, it is necessary to interact effectively within diverse teams and apply the principles of team dynamics. This requires the ability to work collaboratively across professional boundaries and to engage in practices that promote a cooperative and coordinated approach to patient and community care [38].

Interprofessional communication: Health professionals must communicate with sensitivity and responsibility that supports a team approach for the promotion, and maintenance of health, prevention of illnesses, and treatment, with patients, their families, communities, and professionals in health and other fields. This involves effective communication strategies that facilitate collaboration and understanding among diverse healthcare team members, ensuring that care is patient-centered and that health outcomes are optimized [38].

Lifelong Learner: This competency highlights the ability of individuals to keep their knowledge up to date and to remain open to learning at all stages of their lives. Interprofessional education plays a critical role in this area because it enables the integration of knowledge and skills from various disciplines. This integration enhances learning capabilities in a way that allows individuals to solve complex problems they may encounter throughout their careers and to develop innovative solutions. Health professionals should be able to integrate their professional competencies, encompassing continuous professional development and lifelong learning, with interprofessional learning and daily work routines [31].

Collaborative Leadership: Collaborative practice is where health workers from diverse professional backgrounds work together with patients, their families, caregivers, and communities to deliver the highest level of care. In such teamwork, the presence of a leader to manage team dynamics is essential, and the leader can come from any profession. Interprofessional collaboration is a fundamental part of the competencies for health professionals, requiring the ability to collaborate within a framework of skills such as trust, respect, and shared decision-making with colleagues and those from other health professions. The existence of trust and open communication channels among health professionals plays a crucial role in ensuring patient safety and is important in determining a leader during collaboration. This collaboration should be considered from a broad perspective, not only among health workers but also including patients and their families, encompassing all individuals in the health system and society [2, 41–44].

Patient Relations, Recognizing Needs: Placing the patient's needs and beneficial situations at the center of collaborative work requires approaching patients, their families, healthcare providers, and communities as stakeholders in a patient-centered health management system. This emphasizes the importance of understanding and responding to the individual needs of patients, ensuring that care is tailored to their specific circumstances and preferences. It calls for a commitment to actively listen and engage with patients and their support networks to make informed decisions that reflect the best interests of the patient [38, 41–44].

In alignment with these competency areas, scenarios are to be prepared by the workshop managers for the next session.

6.1.1.4 Session 4: creating patient scenarios in accordance with the planned core competencies and competencies

Sharing the prepared sample scenario (20 min).

Working on scenarios (40 min).

This session allowed participants to develop their skills in creating effective patient scenarios in line with the planned core competencies and attributes and provided a valuable resource for use in interprofessional education.

A discussion was held on the scenario examples shared with the trainers participating in the workshop. The scenarios prepared by the nurses working in the Department of Medical Education, Public Health, Family Medicine and Emergency Health Services and Teaching in Nursing with the support of the literature were developed by ensuring the suitability of these scenarios for our country and our university education program due to the differences in the roles and responsibilities of health workers involved in health service delivery according to countries and regions, differences in the health workers represented and cultural differences.

After various reviews of the patient safety scenarios, 40 min session was conducted by the lecturers to ensure content validity. It included the implementation of patient safety IPE, observations, feedback, debriefing, and facilitation.

In these sessions, the trainers identified the important areas in terms of their own professions, especially the boundaries that need to be discussed, the points where professions overlap with each other, positive and negative features, and examples of scenarios suitable for the knowledge and skills that students should gain in line with the competencies determined in this session in the workshop.

6.1.1.5 Session 5: designing assessment tools for scenarios

Success Criteria and Evaluation; After determining the success criteria of scenario-based learning methods in interprofessional education, they should be evaluated effectively [14]. In this section, methods and evaluation criteria that can be used to assess student achievement are discussed. The assessment-evaluation process aims to determine to what extent the objectives set in the design phase of the program have been achieved. The measurement tools to be used in the assessment-evaluation process are determined in advance. The assessment tools, in which the developed scenarios and rubrics will be used, are designed to objectively measure the skills, knowledge, and attitudes gained by the students.

Following the creation of the scenarios, a consensus was reached with the faculty members participating in the workshop in accordance with the scenario within the framework of the competency areas for the previously compiled assessment-evaluation form used to measure the knowledge and skill gains targeted in scenario-based learning programs in the literature. Accordingly, standardization studies were carried out for the seven basic skills assessment sections, sub-headings of each basic skill heading, and scaling for each core competency area.

6.1.1.6 Session 6: evaluation and closing

At the end of the workshop, a closing speech is given by the program managers. In this speech, an overview of the workshop is presented and the contributions of the participants are acknowledged.

Four scenarios covering all core competency areas were developed in the Interprofessional Education Programme booklet. **Table 3** shows the sample scenario, competency areas, and reflection questions.

Home Healthcare Services
Educator:
Facilitator:
Team members: Nutrition Tooth Physiotherapy Nursing Medicine
Competences expected to be gained • roles-responsibilities • relationships with the patient, recognizing their needs • Interprofessional communication • ethical-values • team and teamwork • lifelong learning • collaborative leadership
Scenario: Ayşe Ünlü, a 75-year-old woman with diabetes, was diagnosed with type 2 diabetes 8 years ago. Her blood sugar control is variable and her weight fluctuates a lot. Ayşe, who lives alone, had a total hip replacement operation 3 months ago due to a hip fracture and a physiotherapist comes to her home regularly for exercise. During one of her visits, the physiotherapist noticed a wound on Ayşe's left heel. Seeing that the wound is gradually increasing, she calls the home health unit and asks for the patient to be evaluated in this respect. The physician in charge of the home health unit, who arrived in accordance with his appointment, made the initial examination of the patient, planned the wound care, and stated that he would refer a nutritionist for sugar regulation and a nurse for wound care. In the following days, the nutritionist receives the information about the patient from the physician due to the intensity of her appointments and communicates the nutrition list and recommendations to the patient through the nurse. The nurse visits Ayşe for regular wound care and observes that the wound does not close despite the dressings. Mrs. Ayşe then applies a homemade mixture prepared by her neighbor to her foot. The nurse becomes aware of this situation and the physiotherapist who comes to rehabilitation warns the nurse to inform the physician. The nurse decides to follow the patient for a while. On the next visit, the nurse sees that the wound has become oozing and the leg is bruised. The nurse informs the physician in charge of the home health unit.
Discussion questions: After reading the scenario to one of the students, create a discussion environment with the following questions. Briefly note the answers to the questions and prepare a 10 minute presentation with the team at the end of the session. 1. Which professional groups are included in the scenario? 2. Describe the roles and responsibilities of each professional group in the scenario? and What are the roles and responsibilities that are done and not done (should be)? 3. When you think according to your own professional group, what did this patient primarily need? What are his/her needs? 4. In order to meet the needs of the patient, which communication between professional groups can be different from the scenario? Sample communication sentences should be requested? 5. List the professional groups in terms of preventing the patient's foot wound from progressing? State your possible cooperation suggestion and why? 6. How do you evaluate the relationships between health professionals in the above scenario? Is there teamwork between them? 7. In your opinion, what should be the distribution of tasks that should be followed in routine in terms of sharing and clarifying roles? 8. How did the above scenario make you feel?

Home Healthcare Services

The trainer is expected to pay attention to the following issues during the scenario discussion.

- Define team structure, roles and responsibilities,
- Ask them what they understand by the word "value" (principles, beliefs, ethics, standards, conscience, virtues...)
- What are professional values?
  - Firstly, do no harm (the motto of patient safety, emphasize the other principle of do not harm colleagues and other health professionals), always act by thinking whether what I am doing or trying to do will harm my colleague or other health personnel.
  - If roles are duplicated, we need to think about how we can best combine our efforts.
  - When working, talking to each other, referring, and discharging patients, use clear language and explanations should be detailed.
  - In case of an inappropriate practice by another health worker, a professional should wonder: why is he/she doing this, why did he/she do it? If in doubt, ask.
  - When you ask a colleague to fulfill a task, explain the purpose of the request.
  - For health professionals who are not aware of their values, challenging others or not knowing others' different or opposing values can lead to potential conflict. If not mentioned in the definition of values, you can include in the discussion words or terms that refer specifically to some real values that health professionals have in common: you can think of professional values such as being fair and kind, being fair, telling the truth, respecting, following the law, being hardworking, helping other people, altruistic, honest, self-confident, putting the patient first, etc.
- Identify barriers to team effectiveness.
- Mutual support ve Collaboration konusunda tartışma ortamı yaratın.
- Draw attention to Interprofessional Communication.
- Emphasize team members who are unable to provide an accurate transmission, and who are unable to communicate as soon as possible.
- Assess the behavior of team members who do not speak up or challenge.
- Emphasize team members who do not listen effectively. Discuss what could happen as a result.
- In this scenario, emphasize the lack of mutual support and the lack of necessary skills.
- Could the lack of clear knowledge of roles and responsibilities, lack of cooperation of team members, lack of a collaborative approach, and unethical behavior of health professionals have caused the patient's wound to become infected?
- What is prioritization? Discuss the task of prioritization in roles and responsibilities.
- Discuss what they think about the ability to ask for consultation, which professional groups can ask for consultation in this case, and how formal consultation should be done. (Emphasize the late consultation skill in the scenario)

Table 3.
Sample scenario template.

7. Conclusion and recommendations

This book chapter emphasizes the importance of scenario-based learning in interprofessional education and discusses the basic principles to be considered in the implementation of this strategy and an example of good practice in scenario development. This learning approach allows the development of critical thinking, communication, and teamwork skills in tackling complex health problems while fostering collaboration between students. As a result, this approach has the potential to create positive impacts on both professional development and patient outcomes. Ongoing research will help us to understand the implications of scenario-based learning in even greater depth and optimize its integration into health education practice.

Acknowledgements

The authors would like to extend their heartfelt gratitude to all individuals and institutions that have contributed to the development and realization of this work. Special thanks are directed toward the workshop participants, whose insights and active engagement have significantly enriched this study. We are particularly grateful to FIT, HS, EŞ, HD, ZS, GÇ, GK, GB, ÖÇÖ, and SÇ for their valuable contributions and dedication to the project. Their involvement has been instrumental in shaping the outcomes of this research. Additionally, we acknowledge the support provided by our respective institutions, which facilitated the environment necessary for our collaborative efforts. This project has benefited from the diverse perspectives and expertise of all those involved, reflecting the interprofessional nature of scenario-based learning in inter-professional education.

Conflict of interest

There is no conflict of interest.

Author details

Aysel Başer[1*], Ömer Faruk Sönmez[2] and Hatice Şahin[3]

1 Faculty of Medicine, Department of Medical Education, Izmir Democracy University, Izmir, Turkiye

2 School of Medicine and Population Health, Sheffield, UK

3 Faculty of Medicine, Department of Medical Education, Ege University, Izmir, Turkiye

*Address all correspondence to: aysel.baser@idu.edu.tr

References

[1] Barr H, Norrie C. Requirements Regarding Interprofessional Education and Practice: A Comparative Review for Health and Social Care. [Internet]. Social Work. 2010 [cited 2024 Jun 8]. Available from: https://www.caipe.org/resources/publications/archived-publications/caipe-2010-requirements-regarding-interprofessional-education-and-practice-a-comparative-review-for-health-and-social-care-authored-by-barr-h-norrie-c

[2] Barr H, Gray R, Helme M, Low H, Reeves S. Interprofessional Education Guidelines 2016 Prepared for CAIPE by [Internet]. Vol. 1. Fareham; 2016. Available from: https://www.caipe.org/resources/publications/caipe-publications/barr-h-gray-r-helme-m-low-h-reeves-s-2016-interprofessional-education-guidelines

[3] Menard P, Varpio L. Selecting an interprofessional education model for a tertiary health care setting. Journal of Interprofessional Care. 2014;**28**(4):311-316

[4] Barr H. Competent to collaborate: Towards a competency-based model for interprofessional education. Journal of Interprofessional Care. 1998;**12**(2):181-187

[5] Rossler KL, Kimble LP. Capturing readiness to learn and collaboration as explored with an interprofessional simulation scenario: A mixed-methods research study. Nurse Education Today. 2016;**36**:348-353. Available from: https://pubmed.ncbi.nlm.nih.gov/26363963/

[6] Grosser J, Bientzle M, Kimmerle J. A literature review on the foundations and potentials of digital teaching scenarios for interprofessional health care education. International Journal of Environmental Research and Public Health. 2020;**17**:MDPI AG

[7] Brewer ML, Barr H. Interprofessional education and practice guide No. 8: Team-based interprofessional practice placements. Journal of Interprofessional Care. 2016;**30**(6):747-753. Available from: https://pubmed.ncbi.nlm.nih.gov/27797631/

[8] Hur HK, Kim KK, Lim YM, Kim J, Park KH, Park YC. Patient safety interprofessional education program using medical error scenarios for undergraduate nursing and medical students in Korea. Journal of Interprofessional Care. 2023;**37**(6):944-953. Available from: https://pubmed.ncbi.nlm.nih.gov/36883789/ [Accessed: February 6, 2024]

[9] Michaelsen L, Sweet M, Parmelee D. Team-Based Learning for Health Professions Education: A Guide to Using Small Groups for Improving Learning. John Wiley & Sons; 2011

[10] Buhse M, Della Ratta C. Enhancing interprofessional education with team-based learning. Nurse Educator. 2017;**42**(5):240-244

[11] Lairamore C, George-Paschal L, McCullough K, Grantham M, Head D. A case-based interprofessional education forum increases health students' perceptions of collaboration. The Journal of the International Association of Medical Science Educators. 2013;**23**(3S):472-481

[12] Fox L, Onders R, Hermansen-Kobulnicky CJ, Nguyen TN, Myran L, Linn B, et al. Teaching interprofessional teamwork skills to health professional students: A scoping review. Journal of

Interprofessional Care. 2018;**32**(2): 127-135. Available from: https://www.tandfonline.com/doi/abs/10.1080/13561820.2017.1399868

[13] Scott Reeves HB. Twelve steps to evaluating interprofessional education. Journal of Taibah University Medical Sciences. 2016;**11**(6):601-605

[14] Bahattab A, Caviglia M, Martini D, Hubloue I, Della Corte F, Ragazzoni L. Scenario-based e-simulation Design for Global Health Education: Theoretical foundation and practical recommendations. Journal of Medical Internet Research. 30 Oct 2023;**25**: e46639. Available from: https://www.jmir.org/2023/1/e46639

[15] Drynan D, Murphy S. Understanding anf Faciliating Interproffessional Education: A Guide to Incorporating Interprofessional Experiences into the Practice Education Setting [Internet]. Toronto; 2013. Available from: http://physicaltherapy.med.ubc.ca/files/2012/09/IPE-Guide-2nd-ed.-May-2012.pdf

[16] Spaniol MJ, Rowland NJ. Defining scenario. Futures & Foresight Science. 2019;**1**(1):e3. Available from: https://onlinelibrary.wiley.com/doi/full/10.1002/ffo2.3

[17] Reime MH, Aarflot M, Kvam FI. Does interprofessional scenario-based simulation training change attitudes towards interprofessional learning – A pretest-Posttest study. Journal of Multidisciplinary Healthcare. 2022;**15**: 1527-1532. Available from: https://www.tandfonline.com/action/journalInformation?journalCode=djmd20

[18] Gavilanes JS, An E. Types of Healthcare Simulation: Locations and Training – Who, What, and Where? In: Crawford S, Baily L, Monks S, editors. Comprehensive Healthcare Simulation: Operations, Technology, and Innovative Practice. Cham: Springer; 2019. pp. 13–25

[19] Moro C, Phelps C. Encouraging study in health sciences. Simulation in Healthcare: The Journal of the Society for Simulation in Healthcare. 31 May 2023:37255339

[20] Vaughn J, Erichsen T, Peck J, Arms T, Merryman B, DuBois C, et al. Engaging student learners in interprofessional simulations using Halloween-themed scenarios. Health, Interprofessional Practice and Education. 2023;**5**(0). Available from: https://hipe-pub.org/articles/10.7710/2641-1148.2276

[21] Çelik G, Sönmez ÖF, Başer A. Enhancing interprofessional education readiness in undergraduate dental students: A scenario-based peer learning programme. BMC Oral Health [Internet]. 2024;**24**(1):1-8. Available from: https://bmcoralhealth.biomedcentral.com/articles/10.1186/s12903-024-03878-7 [Accessed: March 12, 2024]

[22] Knowles ME. The Modern Practice of Adult Education. Cambridge: Prentice Hall; 1980. pp. 57-58

[23] Tong S. Active Learning: Theory and Applications. Stanford University; 2001

[24] Kolb DA. Experiential Learning. NJ: Prentice Hall, Englewood Cliffs; 1984

[25] Hean S, Craddock D, Hons MA. Learning theories and interprofessional education: A user's guide. Learning in Health and Social Care. 2009;**8**(4):250-262

[26] Thistlethwaite JE. Values-Based Interprofessional Collaborative Practice: Working Together in Health Care. Cambridge University Press; 2012

[27] Murphy MD, Day DR. A scenario for writing creative scenarios. Socio-Economic Practice and Research. 2021;**3** (2):207-223

[28] Elçin M. A simulation-enhanced, workplace-based interprofessional education for patient safety: Hacettepe University undergraduate experience. Social Innovations Journal. 2020. Available from: https://socialinnovationsjournal.com/index.php/sij/article/view/442/382

[29] Oandasan I, Reeves S. Key elements for interprofessional education. Part 1: The learner, the educator and the learning context. Journal of Interprofessional Care. 2005;**19**(sup1): 23-38

[30] Xavier NA, Brown MR. Interprofessional education in a simulation setting. StatPearls. 2022. Available from: https://www.ncbi.nlm.nih.gov/books/NBK557471/

[31] World Health Organization. Framework for Action on Interprofessional Education & Collaborative Practice Health Professions Networks Nursing & Midwifery Human Resources for Health. 2010. Available from: http://www.who.int/hrh/nursing_midwifery/en/

[32] Yükseköğretim Kurulu (YÖK). YÖK Ulusal Çekirdek Eğitim Programı. 2022. Available from: https://www.yok.gov.tr/kurumsal/idari-birimler/egitim-ogretim-dairesi/ulusal-cekirdek-egitimi-programlari

[33] Yükseköğretim Kurulu (YÖK). YÖK Ulusal Çekirdek Eğitim Programı_ Hemşirelik Ulusal Çekirdek Eğitim Programı (HUÇEP). 2014. Available from: https://www.yok.gov.tr/kurumsal/idari-birimler/egitim-ogretim-dairesi/ulusal-cekirdek-egitimi-programlari

[34] Yükseköğretim Kurulu (YÖK). YÖK Ulusal Çekirdek Eğitim Programı_ Fizyoterapi ve Rehabilitasyon Ulusal Çekirdek Eğitim Programı. 2016. Available from: https://www.yok.gov.tr/kurumsal/idari-birimler/egitim-ogretim-dairesi/ulusal-cekirdek-egitimi-programlari

[35] Yükseköğretim Kurulu (YÖK). YÖK Ulusal Çekirdek Eğitim Programı_ Beslenme ve Diyetetik Ulusal Çekirdek Eğitim Programı. 2016. Available from: https://www.yok.gov.tr/kurumsal/idari-birimler/egitim-ogretim-dairesi/ulusal-cekirdek-egitimi-programlari

[36] Yükseköğretim Kurulu (YÖK). YÖK Ulusal Çekirdek Eğitim Programı_ Mezuniyet Öncesi Diş Hekimliği Eğitimi Ulusal Çekirdek Eğitim Programı (DUÇEP). 2016.

[37] Yükseköğretim Kurulu (YÖK). Mezuniyet Öncesi Tıp Eğitimi Ulusal Çekirdek Programı. Ulusal Çekirdek Eğitim Programı. 2020;**2021**. Available from: https://www.yok.gov.tr/kurumsal/idari-birimler/egitim-ogretim-dairesi/ulusal-cekirdek-egitimi-programlari

[38] Interprofessional Education Collaborative (IPEC). Core Competencies for Interprofessional Collaborative Practice: 2016 Update. 2016

[39] Buring SM, Westberg S, Broeseker A, Hansen L, Bhushan A, Duncan-Hewitt W, et al. Interprofessional education: Definitions, student competencies, and guidelines for implementation. American Journal of Pharmaceutical Education. 2011;**73**(4): 59. Available from: https://www.ajpe.org/doi/pdf/10.5688/aj730459

[40] Wood V, Flavell A, Vanstolk D, Bainbridge L, Nasmith L. The road to collaboration: Developing an

interprofessional competency framework. Journal of Interprofessional Care. 2009;**23**(6):621-629. Available from: https://www.tandfonline.com/action/journalInformation?journalCode=ijic20

[41] Canadian Interprofessional Health Collaborative (CIHC). A National Interprofessional Competency Framework. Canada; 2010. Available from: www.cihc.ca

[42] Interprofessional Education Collaborative (IPEC). Core Competencies for Interprofessional Collaborative Practice: Report of an Expert Panel. Washington DC: Interprofessional Education Collaborative; 2011. p. 1351. Available from: http://www.ncbi.nlm.nih.gov/pubmed/22030650

[43] Thistlethwaite JE, Forman D, Matthews LR, Rogers GD, Steketee C, Yassine T. Competencies and frameworks in interprofessional education: A comparative analysis. Academic Medicine. 2014;**89**(6):869-875

[44] World Health Organization (WHO). Working Together for Health. 2006. Available from: https://apps.who.int/iris/handle/10665/43432

Chapter 6

Triple Taxon Test/Technique: An Innovative Method for Self-Learning and Self-Evaluation in Health Problems

Seyed Mansour Razavi, Mehdi Afkar and Parisa Shojaei

Abstract

To manage a patient, physicians, and medical students need to collect the patient's data and information in different ways, evaluate, interpret, analyze clinical reasoning, and, after diagnosis, take action to solve the patient's problem. For this purpose, they must pass at least three summarized categories of the cognition domain. These three categories include: remembering, interpretation, and problem-solving. In this article, we intend to introduce an innovative case-based practice or test technique to our audiences, which includes all three above-mentioned categories. We have named this method TTT (Triple Taxonomy Tests/technique) or MTQ (Mixed Taxonomy Questions). This form of case-based test/technique is applicable in self-learning, self-assessment, or official evaluations, which is explained below in the form of an example.

Keywords: problem-based learning, self-assessment, conversion disorder, mass hysteria, medical students

1. Introduction

Psychologists have divided educational fields into three categories, including "cognitive," "emotional," and "psychomotor" domains. Benjamin Bloom has classified the field of cognition from the lowest level (remembering) to the highest level (evaluation and creation) [1, 2].

Medical sciences teachers must use higher levels of these three domains to improve the quality of students' learning and not be limited only to the lower levels, particularly in the cognitive domain. The quality of learning of medical students may decline without targeting higher cognitive levelsof abilities such as evaluation, interpretation, analysis, reasoning, and creation [3]. Therefore, medical students are expected to learn such high-level cognitive skills [4], and acquiring these abilities is vital for their future performance [3].

The importance of active involvement of medical students in clinical issues is generally accepted by medical education experts for improving the quality of learning, and various methods are used to achieve this goal. Understanding this need has led medical schools to adopt and implement some degrees of integration of basic and clinical sciences (vertical integration). The use of clinical cases to help teaching, which is called case-based learning (CBL), is one of the most interesting strategies in this field, and different types of implementations of this method have been described [5, 6].

On the other hand, lifelong learning skills, including self-learning and self-assessment, are also among the most important strategies accepted in adult education and vital for the professional development of doctors. Case-based questions are one of the useful tools that can be used in the field of self-learning and self-evaluation by students in the teaching and learning process [7, 8].

Also, one of the important components of the educational process is measuring the educational progress of learners and evaluating their quality of learning. Several research have been conducted about the quality of exams held in universities and higher education institutions. The results of many of these studies have shown that many teachers enter the field of teaching without getting enough training in measuring methods and designing tests. As well as, most of the findings of these studies have shown that the teachers, to measure students' academic progress, often emphasize superficial and simple concepts, and many times, the questions are ambiguous and are not purposeful [9].

The results of Josefowicz's study showed that teachers spent a lot of time preparing course materials, but they did not spend much time designing exam questions, and their knowledge of evaluation principles and exam question design techniques was insufficient [10]. The available evidence shows that training faculty members and giving them appropriate feedback have improved the quality of exam questions, especially multiple-choice questions, and improved student evaluation conditions [11].

To improve the quality of students' learning and encourage them to think and act at different levels of the cognitive domain, we have invented a new case-based method, which we introduce in this present article.

The purpose of this article is to encourage students to make logical use of what they have learned, practice, and strengthen the ability to interpret, analyze, criticize, clinically reason, diagnose, and solve patients' problems.

2. Introducing TTT (triple taxonomy test/technique)

Three-level case-based questions or TTT (Triple Taxon Test/Technique) and dual-purpose questions are designed questions in the field of patient management, and medical students can use them for self-study and self-evaluation to strengthen their professional capabilities in three categories of "remembering", "interpretation and reasoning," and "olvingsroblem-p". On this occasion, we intend to present one of these cases to the audience to get familiar with this technique or test.

3. Case features

- They are placement test questions.
- They are case-based and practical questions.
- They include the taxonomies of recall, interpretation, and problem-solving.

DOI: http://dx.doi.org/10.5772/intechopen.114071

- They contain a trunk with several blank spaces.
- They contain several characteristic, contradictory, or unrelated options.
- The score of each space is one, and the value coefficient of the questions is the same.
- Students will receive a lot of information in the feedback of these questions.

4. How to design a case

- We choose a real case, among the numerous interesting clinical cases.
- We specify the questions in three categories of *recall*, *interpretation,* and *problem-solving*.
- Inside the case, we remove the keywords and replace them with blank spaces.
- In the *remembering* section, we use options that the examinee can only use his / her memory to select those options.
- In the *interpretation* section, we use options whose selection requires interpretation, reasoning, calculation, analysis, comparison, use of standards (cut-off points), and diagnosis.
- And in the decision-making and *problem-solving* section, we choose options that are helpful for diagnosis and treatment, development, judgment, selection, and problem-solving.
- We arrange the options under the case description.
- It should be noted that for each answer option, there must be a valid reference.
- Among the options, we have also included the correct option (the main answer to the question), prepositions, and contradictory words.
- The feedback section to the students is completed with the instructor's explanations and using authentic sources.

5. Introducing an example of TTT cases

This article presents an innovative case-based method for better learning for medical students. With this method, it is possible to design tens, hundreds, and thousands of cases of common diseases. In this case, our main contacts are medical interns, faculty members, and assistants in internal medicine, infectious diseases, social and family medicine, pediatrics, adult and child psychiatry, adult and child neurology, clinical psychology, health psychology, and medical education.

6. Notice to the audience

Dear audience, please first read the case carefully and fill in the blanks using the options below, give yourself a grade, then by reading the answers, assess your abilities in the three areas of "remembering," "reasoning and interpretation," and "problem-solving." (The maximum score in this case is 16).

7. Case presentation

In the interval between the two national days of the Polio Mass Vaccination plan to eradicate polio, in 1994 AD (equal to 1373s), in Ahmedabad village, Ardakan township, Yazd province, in Iran, a sudden incident occurred with paralysis in the upper limbs of two 12- and 13-year-old girls of a middle school. Then, within a week, the disease spread to 15 other students of the same school, all of whom were 12 years old. At the same time, four other students who were 9 years old from an elementary school near the first high school were diagnosed with upper limb paralysis. (A total of 21 students).

The onset of the disease was at the same time as national and regional advertisements about the necessity of vaccination against polio and explaining the consequences of lack of vaccination among people. National days were held in the months of April and May (near the final exams of the students) [12].

Immediately after confirming the ...., among these students, all of them were evaluated separately by specialized medical teams, including pediatricians, infectious disease experts, neurologists, and psychologists. The schools were temporarily closed. The village environment and schools were also evaluated by environmental health experts and entomologists, and the necessary measures were taken.

The socioeconomic status of the affected girls was low to medium, and the average family size was six people; the occupation of most of the household heads was agriculture and animal husbandry. The .... was a 13-year-old girl, taller than her classmates, who had failed in the last class for 1 year.

According to the records, vaccination of all affected girls except one of them was complete against diseases, especially poliomyelitis. The signs and symptoms of the disease in the vast majority of patients were in the form of paralysis of the right upper limb (except for one of the girls who was left-handed, and her left hand was paralyzed); pain in the joints of fingers, wrists, and elbows; and muscle pain during passive movements of the limb. All of them had disturbances of sensation, touch, heat, itching, and marked paresthesia in the affected limb, and in most cases, there was also headache and anorexia.

In clinical examinations, the patients did not have a fever or skin lesions, the reflexes of the organs were relatively normal, and, psychologically, they were very anxious, and some of them had a history of stuttering, anxiety, nightmare, feeling homesickness, depression, and sleep disorders, and the symptoms were reduced or disappeared with a brief dictation (to suggest).

No special problems were found in environmental health inspections. And there was found in entomological assessments of the schools, houses, animal shelters, etc. A significant number of .... that this indicated the possibility of tick paralysis.

According to the obtained data and information, specialists suggested ...., ..., ..., epidemic polyarthritis (Ross river fever), clinical features caused by arboviruses, and psychiatric disorders such as .... for the patients, and they requested the necessary diagnostic tests for the main diagnosis.

In the performed tests, blood cell count, sedimentation rate, CRP, liver function tests, peripheral blood smear for Borrelia Burgdorferi spirochetes, urine analysis, polio screening tests, electrodiagnostic tests, and joint proceedings were all normal.

Without any action, by temporarily closing schools, during the summer, all the girls recovered, and the wave of the disease subsided, and the patients were only monitored. With the arrival of October and the reopening of schools, the disease among several middle school girls (including the index case) recurred. To solve this problem, experts suggested ....

The points that did not confirm the existence of an organic communicable disease, especially poliomyelitis, were:

The completeness of the vaccination of most of the affected girls against polio; the rarity of .... and .... in polio; the absence of infection in the community, especially among family members; lack of skin lesions caused by insect bites, especially ticks; and the absence of ticks on any part of the body of the affected students. Absence of arthritis in the majority of sufferers (among the sufferers, joint problems were mostly in the form of arthralgia, except for two cases who also had mild arthritis); lack of .... appearance on the skin, which is a characteristic sign for Lyme disease, absence of fever; maculopapular rashes; and bilateral arthritis; which all rule out the disease of .... and the absence of any evidence of organic diseases, especially infections in the performed para-clinical tests.

The points that confirmed the existence of mass hysteria consisted of:

The patients rewe female (mass hysteria is more common in females). This disorder is more common in .... societies, and sufferers of this disorder ....

The character of the case index is of interest and attraction to the others, and she dominates her peers intellectually, and she is a role model for her classmates and causes .... The dominant hand of all sufferers indicates a symbolic connection. The existence of .... advertisements against polio and, at the same time, the stress of end-of-year exams are also effective factors, and finally, the recovery of those affected after being encouraged to compete in volleyball as a team is a determining factor [12]. Score: 16.

Options:

endemic - epidemic - outbreak- cluster- health problem - Primary case - Index case- mosquitos - mites - hard tick Ixodes scapularis - bedbugs - Poliomyelitis - Tick paralysis - Mosquito bite arthralgia - Bedbug bite syndrome - Lead poisoning - mass hysteria - Lyme disease - Conducting a course of physiotherapy - prescribing corticosteroids - organizing a movement competition such as volleyball - closing school - paresthesia - Motor reflex disorder - sensory disorder - Bull's eye - petechial - infectious arthritis - Ross river fever - animal husbandry jobs – a high socioeconomic level more than the community where they live - low to medium socioeconomic level - pre-puberty - think logically - have high self-esteem - are very suggestible - assimilation - bad education caused by - stress caused by.

8. Answers to case questions

8.1 Please check your answers once again before viewing the answers

In the interval between the two national days of the Polio Mass Vaccination plan to eradicate polio, in 1994 AD (equal to 1373s), in Ahmedabad village, Ardakan township, Yazd province, in Iran, a sudden incident occurred with paralysis in the upper limbs of two 12- and 13-year-old girls of a middle school. Then, within a week, the disease spread to 15 other students of the same school, all of whom were 12 years old. At the same time, four other students who were 9 years old from an elementary school near the first high school were diagnosed with upper limb paralysis. (A total of 21 students).

The onset of the disease was at the same time as national and regional advertisements about the necessity of vaccination against polio and explaining the consequences of lack of vaccination among people. National days were held in the months of April and May (near the final exams of the students) [12].

Immediately after confirming the *health problem* among these students, all of them were evaluated separately by specialized medical teams, including pediatricians, infectious disease experts, neurologists, and psychologists. The schools were temporarily closed. The village environment and schools were also evaluated by environmental health experts and entomologists, and the necessary measures were taken.

The socioeconomic status of the affected girls was low to medium, and the average family size was six people, the occupation of most of the household heads was agriculture and animal husbandry. The *index case* was a 13-year-old girl, taller than her classmates, who had failed in the last class for a year.

According to the records, vaccination of all affected girls except one of them was complete against diseases, especially poliomyelitis. The signs and symptoms of the disease in the vast majority of patients were in the form of paralysis of the right upper limb (except for one of the girls who was left-handed, and her left hand was paralyzed); pain in the joints of fingers, wrists, and elbow; and muscle pain during passive movements of the limb. All of them had disturbances of sensation, touch, heat, itching, and marked paresthesia in the affected limb, and in most cases, there was also headache and anorexia.

In clinical examinations, the patients did not have a fever or skin lesions, the reflexes of the organs were relatively normal, and psychologically, they were very anxious, and some of them hada history of stuttering, anxiety, nightmare, feeling homesickness, depression, and sleep disorders, and the symptoms were reduced or disappeared with a brief dictation (to suggest).

No special problems were found in environmental health inspections. And there was found in entomological assessments of the schools, houses, animal shelters, etc. A significant number of *hard tick Ixodes scapularis* indicated the possibility of tick paralysis.

According to the obtained data and information, specialists suggested *Poliomyelitis, Tick paralysis, Lyme disease*, epidemic polyarthritis (Ross river fever), clinical features caused by arboviruses, and psychiatric disorders such as *mass hysteria* for the patients, and they requested the necessary diagnostic tests for the main diagnosis.

In the performed tests, blood cell count, sedimentation rate, CRP, liver function tests, peripheral blood smear for Borrelia Burgdorferi spirochetes, urine analysis, polio screening tests, electrodiagnostic tests, and joint proceedings were all normal.

Without any action, temporarily closing schools, during the summer, all the girls recovered, and the wave of the disease subsided, and the patients were only monitored. With the arrival of October and the reopening of schools, the disease among several middle school girls (including the index case) recurred. To solve this problem, experts suggested *organizing a movement competition such as volleyball.*

The points that did not confirm the existence of an organic communicable disease, especially poliomyelitis, were:

The completeness of the vaccination of most of the affected girls against polio; the rarity of *paresthesia* and *sensory disorder* in polio; the absence of infection in the community, especially among family members; lack of skin lesions caused by insect bites, especially ticks; and the absence of ticks on any part of the body of the affected students. Absence of arthritis in the majority of sufferers (among the sufferers, joint problems were mostly in the form of arthralgia, except for two cases who also had mild arthritis), lack of *Bull's-eye appearance* on the skin, which is a characteristic sign for Lyme disease, absence of fever, macule popular rashes, and bilateral arthritis, which all rule out the disease of *Ross River Fever* and the absence of any evidence of organic diseases, especially infections in the performed para-clinical tests.

The points that confirmed the existence of mass hysteria consisted of:

The patients rewe female (mass hysteria is more common in females). This disorder is more common in *low to medium socioeconomic level* societies, and sufferers of this disorder *are very suggestible.*

The character of the case index is of interest and attraction to the others, and she dominates her peers intellectually, and she is a role model for her classmates and causes *assimilation.* The dominant hand of all sufferers indicates a symbolic connection. The existence of *stress caused by* advertisements against polio and, at the same time, the stress of end-of-year exams are also effective factors, and finally, the recovery of those affected after being encouraged to compete in volleyball as a team is a determining factor [12]. Score: 16.

9. Discussion/feedback

Here we discuss the above case, in the Remembering, Interpretation, and Problem-solving domains. Here, after the students have thought about the case in the allotted time, we give them feedback in the above three areas.

9.1 Remembering

- *What do you know about Mass Vaccination Polio in Iran?*

In 1988, the World Health Organization (WHO) suggested the strategy of mass vaccination to countries on national days [13]. The first efforts to eradicate polio in Iran started in the 1950s, but it did not succeed because it was not accompanied by universal vaccination. This problem continued, and it took victims especially in remote border towns and villages until an important incident happened inthe 1373s. Basij volunteer forces, with the help of the Ministry of Health, did important work with coordinated action [14].

More than 320,000 Basij volunteers vaccinated about nine million children under the age of five all over Iran against polio in just one day. In this project, the Basij parties formed more than 175,000 relief groups (auxiliary groups) in 16,000 vaccination centers, and eventually polio was eradicated in Iran. The effect of the work was so surprising that, in the same year, a letter was written to the President of Iran by UNISE, who was thanked for this important action. In this letter, it was mentioned that "Iran is the only country in the world where health indicators were improved during the war and there were no deaths caused by infectious diseases." Fortunately, polio has been eradicated in Iran since 1374 [14].

- *In the above case, was the 13* year- *year old girl an index case or a primary case? What is the difference between these two terms?*

An index case is the first patient identified and reported by health authorities, and a primary case is a person who brings the disease to the community, school, another person, or even the country, and in most cases, it remains unknown [15]. So, the 13–year-old girl, for the first time, before performing any interventions is the index case.

- *What are the differential diagnoses of paralysis?*

Poliomyelitis, tick-borne paralysis, Lyme disease, Ross River disease, Hysteria, and so on.

- *What is the cause of tick-borne paralysis?*

Ixodes scapularis blood-sucking tick toxin.

Tick paralysis is a relatively rare and fatal disease caused by some blood-sucking species of female ticks from the Ixodidae family, especially Dermacentor andersoni and Ixodes scapularis. This disease, which is characterized by acute ascending flaccid paralysis, is usually misdiagnosed with other neurological diseases, especially Guillain-Barré syndrome, due to similar clinical manifestations [16].

- *What is mass hysteria?*

Mass hysteria or widespread hysteria (Epidemic Hysteria) is a manifestation of a conversion disorder that often occurs when people in a society are simultaneously under a stressor. This type of conversion disorder occurs in different clinical forms, including limb paralysis [12].

- *Which of the symptoms in affected girls is not common in polio?*

Paresthesia and sensory disturbance [12].

- *What is Ross River fever?*

Ross River fever is an epidemic polyarthritis that is transmitted by mosquitoes, and fever, fatigue, skin rashes, pain and swelling of the joints are symptoms of the disease and may last for several weeks to several months [17].

- *What are Lyme disease and its characteristic sign?*

Lyme disease is caused by a spirochete named Borrelia Burgdorferi. This bacterium is transmitted to humans through the bite of infected black-legged ticks. Typical symptoms include fever, headache, fatigue, and a characteristic skin rash called erythema migrants [18]. Skin rashes are a common symptom of Lyme disease. Cutaneous manifestations are usually seen as a single circle that slowly spreads from the tick bite site. It may be marked in the center and look like a target board or "Bull's eye sign." This characteristic rash is often warm to the touch but usually not painful or itchy [18].

9.2 Interpretation

- *Immediately after confirming what were all of the affected girls visited by specialized teams? Why did not you choose other options?*

Because, at this stage, the various aspects of the case have not yet been clarified, the best word that is suggested for this situation is "health problem." In explaining why, it is better not to use the other words, we refer to the specific definitions of the words given in the options below.

The occurrence of more than the "expected limit" of a disease, an event, or special behavior, compared to the normal state, in the same region, same population, and in the same season of the year, is called an epidemic [19]. The records showed that there were no such situations in the region.

The outbreak has the same definition as an epidemic, but it is often used for a limited geographic area and is more related to an infectious disease [19]. In this stage, it is not yet clear whether the cases are infectious or not.

A disease is said to be endemic in a specific region or population, which is stable and continuous in that region [20], and this condition has occurred for the first time in the region and has not existed before.

And finally, the expected accumulation of relatively uncommon events or diseases in an area is called a cluster. Cluster studies are usually used for non-infectious diseases such as cancers, spontaneous abortions, suicide, congenital anomalies, and so on. Cluster studies are also called Small Area Analyzes. The most common design for such studies is the case-control study [19].

- *What diagnoses did the experts make for these patients and why?*

In the situation under discussion, due to the social tensions that were created during the mass vaccination of children under 5 years of age in society and familiesof affected girls, at first, experts should have considered the paralysis caused by the vaccination against polio.

The other diagnoses were: Tick paralysis and Lyme disease, due to the incident in the village and the occupation of the families in animal husbandry, and the presence of some symptoms and mass hysteria due to the observation of certain contradictory behaviors in the patients.

- *What were the reasons that these girls were not affected by polio?*

These reasons are given below:

The reasons that did not confirm the existence of an organic communicable disease, especially polio among affected girls, were:

Completeness of vaccination against poliomyelitis among most of the affected girls. The presence of paresthesia and sensory disturbances in girls' responses to physicians, which are usually not the symptoms of polio. The contradiction of patients' responses to different doctors. Absence of similar diseases among the community members, especially the family members of the patients. Lack of skin lesions that were contrary to insect bites, especially ticks, and not seeing ticks anywhere on the affected 'girls bodies. Absence of arthritis in the majority of the patients (among the patients, joint problems were mostly in the form of arthralgia, except in two cases who also had mild arthritis). The absence of a Bull's-eye appearance on the skin is a characteristic sign of Lyme disease. Absence of fever, maculopapular rashes, and bilateral arthritis rules out Ross River Fever, and absence of signs of organic diseases, especially infectious diseases, in performed para-clinical tests [12].

- *What are the reasons which confirm that these girls are suffering from mass hysteria?*

The points that confirmed the existence of collective hysteria were: the patients being female (mass hysteria is more common in females). This disorder is more common in the low to middle socioeconomic levels of society. And sufferers of this disorder are psychologically suggestible.

The index case is the center of attention of her friends and other persons. She has an intellectual superiority over them and is a role model for them. This feature causes them to be assimilated. The dominant hand of all patients indicates a symbolic connection. As well as, the presence of stress caused by advertisements against polio disease and, at the same time, the stress of end-of-year exams is also an effective factor [20].

- *Now that the diagnosis is known, which of the words, endemic, epidemic, outbreak, or cluster, do you choose for this phenomenon?*

By analyzing the conditions in the above definitions, we choose the word cluster [21].

- *How to determine that the limb is not paralyzed?*

By carefully examining the reflexes of the affected upper limbs. If there is no paralysis, the reflexes are normal. (Normal mode detection).

9.3 Problem-solving

- *What actions were taken for the patients?*

Psychotherapy - moving a paralyzed hand - giving nutritional supplements etc.

- *What actions were taken for the patients with the recurrence of the disease?*

With the diagnosis of mass hysteria, a volleyball competition was organized among the students of several schools in the province, and the affected students were encouraged to participate. In these competitions, it was observed that the students used their hands well in different movement directions without any complaints.

10. Conclusion

We have innovated a new case-based method for self-study, self-assessment, practicing applied topics, and official evaluations of students. We have named this method TTT (Triple Taxonomy Test/technique) or MTQ (Mixed Taxonomy Questions). We hope that our audiences be familiar with this method and test their ability in reasoning, interpretation, and problem-solving.

It is suggested that the respected faculty members of different disciplines prepare a number of these cases from common diseases and use them for the students, according to their academic level (e.g., apprentices, interns, and residents). In our department, we have used this method by evaluating 20 parameters for medical students by designing 10 different cases, and the initial results indicate that the students are welcome; we are waiting to complete the number of samples.

Acknowledgements

We hereby consider it necessary to thank all the respected specialists who tried to diagnose these patients 30 years ago, as well as all the dear girls who are currently the mothers, brides and daughters of our country, and wish them the best for their health in all aspects.

Funding

This study did not receive any specific grant from funding agencies in the public, commercial, or not-for-profit sectors.

Conflict of interest

The authors declare that there is no conflict of interest.

Author details

Seyed Mansour Razavi[1,2*], Mehdi Afkar[3,4] and Parisa Shojaei[3,4]

1 Faculty of Medicine, Tehran Medical Science, Department of Community Medicine, Islamic Azad University, Tehran, Iran

2 Drug Rational Research Center, Tehran University of Medical Sciences and Health Services, Tehran, Iran

3 Faculty of Medicine, Tehran Medical Science, Department of Community and Preventive Medicine, IslamicAzad University, Tehran, Iran

4 Social Determinants of Health Research Center, Tehran Islamic Azad University of Medical Sciences, Tehran, Iran

*Address all correspondence to: shojaee7@gmail.com

References

[1] LasleyII TJ. Bloom's taxonomy: Encyclopedia Britannica. 2023. Available from: https://www.britannica.com/topic/Blooms-taxonomy

[2] Armstrong P. Bloom's Taxonomy Vanderbilt University Center for Teaching: Vanderbilt University, Center for Teaching. 2010 Available from: https://cft.vanderbilt.edu/guides-sub-pages/blooms-taxonomy/

[3] Tuma F, Nassar AK. Applying Bloom's taxonomy in clinical surgery: Practical examples. Annals of Medicine and Surgery. 2021;**69**:102656

[4] Vykhrushch AV, Khvalyboha TI, Fedchyshyn NO, Bagriy M, Fedoniuk L, Protsyk H, et al. Development of medical students creativity as a priority of modern higher education. Wiadomości lekarskie, LXXIV. 2021;**12**:3204-3213

[5] McLean SF. Case-based learning and its application in medical and health-care fields: A review of worldwide literature. Journal of Medical Education and Curricular Development. 2016;**3**:JMECD. S20377

[6] Naeimi L, Alizadeh M, Shariati M. Case based learning: The concept, models, effectiveness and challenges. Journal of Medical Education and Development. 2016;**3**(11):201-209

[7] Reed S, Shell R, Kassis K, Tartaglia K, Wallihan R, Smith K, et al. Applying adult learning practices in medical education. Current Problems in Pediatric and Adolescent Health Care. 2014;**44**(6):170-181

[8] Li S, Yu B, Yue J. Case-oriented self-learning and review in pharmacology teaching. The American Journal of the Medical Sciences. 2014;**348**(1):52-56

[9] Shakurnia A, Khosravi Borojeni A, Mozaffari A, Elhampour H. An evaluation of exam questions designed by faculty members emphasizing on the multiple choice question structure Ahvaz Jundishapur university of medical sciences 2007. Strides in Development of Medical Education. 2010;**6**(2):129-138

[10] Jozefowicz RF, Koeppen BM, Case S, Galbraith R, Swanson D, Glew RH. The quality of in-house medical school examinations. Academic Medicine. 2002;**77**(2):156-161

[11] Mohammadi Zeidi A, Heydarnia A, M K. Comparing test preparation methods in the school of public health before and after test standardization workshop. In: Abstract of the 9th National Congress of Medical Education. Yazd: Yazd University of Medical Sciences; 2008

[12] Harazi MA, Razavi SM. A Case of epidemic hysteria: A Case report. Pejouhesh dar Pezeshki (Research in Medicine). 1997;**21**(3):81-86

[13] Sutter RW, Maher C. Mass vaccination campaigns for polio eradication: An essential strategy for success. Current Topics in Microbiology and Immunology. 2006;**304**:195-220

[14] History of vaccination and diseases that have been controlled, eliminated or eradicated in Iran: Health Services Management. 2020. Available from: https://hcsm.ir/1399/01/

[15] Njogu T. Difference between Index Case and Primary Case. Difference between Similar Terms and Objects. 2021. Available from: http://www.differencebetween.net/miscellaneous/difference-between-index-case-and-primary-case/

[16] Fazeli-Dinan M, Karimi N, Enayati A. Tick paralysis, cause, symptoms, diagnosis and treatment. Journal of Mazandaran University of Medical Sciences. 2016;**26**(138):215-231

[17] Ross River virus disease: National Center for Emerging and Zoonotic Infectious Diseases (NCEZID). 2022. Available from: https://wwwnc.cdc.gov/travel/diseases/ross-river-virus-disease

[18] Lyme disease: Centers for Disease Control and Prevention, National Center for Emerging and Zoonotic Infectious Diseases (NCEZID), Division of Vector-Borne Diseases (DVBD). 2022. Available from: https://www.cdc.gov/lyme/index.html#:~:text=Lyme%20disease%20is%20caused%20by,skin%20rash%20called%20erythema%20migrans

[19] Introduction to Epidemiology: Centers for Disease Control and Prevention, National Center for Emerging and Zoonotic Infectious Diseases (NCEZID), Division of Vector-Borne Diseases (DVBD). 2012. Available from: https://www.cdc.gov/csels/dsepd/ss1978/lesson1/section11.html#:~:text=Epidemic%20refers%20to%20an%20increase,a%20more%20limited%20geographic%20area

[20] Endemic (epidemiology). 2023. Available from: https://en.wikipedia.org/wiki/Endemic_(epidemiology)

[21] Razavi SM. Investigation and Control of Epidemics. Comprehensive Book of Public Health. Principles and Applications of Epidemiology, 4. Tehran: Arjmand; 2019. p. 1287

Chapter 7

Medical Education Technology in Resource-Limited Settings

Pebalo Francis Pebolo, Ayikoru Jackline, Maxwell Opwonya, Raymond Otim and Felix Bongomin

Abstract

The integration of information and communication technology (ICT) in medical education is crucial to meet the evolving needs of the global population and ensure competency among healthcare trainees. In low- and middle-income countries (LMICs), where resources are limited, leveraging advanced ICTs has the potential to revolutionize medical education by promoting student-centred learning through asynchronous and distributed access. The recent introduction of artificial intelligence (AI) = in medical education has transformed learning into a personalized experiences, virtual simulations, and real-time feedback. Our experience with use of simple technology in Uganda serves as a prime example of how innovative technologies are being utilized to enhance medical education in a LMICs setting. Our experience in the implementation of interactive displays in simulation training and the establishment of low-cost content production studio has significantly improved trainings and learnings. By integrating these technologies closer to the learning environment, students can access information before or after interacting with their teachers, engage in higher cognitive activities, and stimulate problem-solving skills. The success of these initiatives demonstrates their potential for adoption to elevate the quality of medical education in LMICs. Embracing ICT in medical training not only bridges educational gaps but also fosters inclusive and equitable access to resources in LMICs.

Keywords: content production studio, medical educational technology in Uganda, simulation training, digital divide, medical training in resource limited settings, interactive screen

1. Introduction

The future medical needs of the ever-growing global population necessitate a significant overhaul in medical education to ensure competency. Efforts should be directed towards promoting student-centred learning methods, which have proven to be more effective than teacher-centred ones. In this era, advancement of information and communication technology (ICT) has proven imperative in offering transformative learning avenues for instance producing, distributing, and accessing educational content [1], including within clinical environments [2]. Despite challenges in resource-limited settings, the adoption of technology holds promise in overcoming barriers to access and enhancing quality of medical education. Use of personal computers, projectors, interactive screens, and the Internet has revolutionized the teaching and learning of medicine. Recent innovations in artificial intelligence, such as machine learning and large language modelling, have presented a challenge to educators, as students can now access knowledge and instructions at their own pace and convenience. This necessitates a shift in the delivery of educational content, requiring educators to focus on application, analysis, evaluation, and creation, as outlined in Bloom's taxonomy [3]. In this chapter, we discuss the use of ICT in medical education and reflect on our experiences in introducing some simple but advanced educational technologies in Ugandan contexts and highlight the reasons for the low uptake of these technologies in low resource settings.

2. Medical education and information and communication technology

The primary aim of most medical education curricula is to ensure the successful achievement of specific learning outcomes, leading to the development of competent students. These achievements heavily depend on finding a balance between the workload and the time available for students [4], as well as the methods of content delivery. ICT is an innovative tool that can be used to make learning active, particularly by fostering student-centeredness integrating it closer to the classroom or clinical patient environment. This allows students to access information before or after interacting with faculties [5]. Moreover, ICT can also be harnessed to create activities that engage students' cognitive processes, ensuring that their natural responses are stimulated to solve problems [6].

Despite the challenges posed by limited resources, medical institutions in low-resource settings have established educational technology or media centres to harness the power of ICT in education. These initiatives aim to bridge the gap between traditional and modern teaching methods, ensuring that students receive quality education regardless of their geographic location or access to technology.

2.1 The digital divide

The fulfilment of technology in education aligns with the United Nation's Sustainable Development Goal (SDG) 4, ensuring inclusive and equitable education and promoting lifelong learning opportunities, despite the absence of a specific target for educational technology in the SDG. The production of accessible educational content without restrictions to institutions or geographic areas help reduce inequality in access to educational resources. Advancements in technology have innovatively enhanced the delivery of curricula in many institutions, promoting more effective learning methods.

Regrettably, not all institutions have the luxury of investing in ICT infrastructures and skilled man powers [7, 8]. Even among those that have heavily invested, not all students or faculties have access to ICT. Additionally, cultural and socioeconomic factors may influence the acceptance and implementation of new technologies [9]. This has resulted into some institutions using more ICT compared to others and among some students with technology privileges compared to others. This creates a digital divide which is the gap between those with and those without access to ICT, a situation particularly evident in LMICs, such as Uganda.

The digital divide in low-income countries can be classified into the following categories. Firstly, there is a divide due to limited or lack of access, where poor students may not have smartphones or personal computers, limiting their access to ICT-related educational contents at their own time, pace, and place. Additionally, divides exist due to lack of or failure to maintain ICT infrastructures. More so, costly and unreliable Internet connectivity further exacerbates the digital divide, affecting distributed and asynchronous access.

Furthermore, there is a divide due to the generational gap, with different generations (X, Y, and Z) bringing unique characteristics and teaching/learning preferences. Generation X (born between 1965 and 1980) [10] may prefer a more independent learning approach and might have challenges using technology, potentially impacting the quality of educational materials they produce if they become educators. Generation Y (born between 1981 and 1996) [10] are often tech-savvy and respond well to interactive and technology-enhanced learning experiences. Many educators belonging to this generation are able to navigate technology and incorporate it into their teaching tools. Generation Z (born between 1997 and 2012) [11] are the true digital natives comfortable with technology from a young age, preferring engaging and visually illustrative ICTs content. Educators can take these generational traits into account when designing curriculum, selecting teaching methods, and incorporating technology into medical education to better meet the needs of learners from each generation.

2.2 Medical education technology

In the ever-evolving field of medical education, the integration of technological advancements is paramount in ensuring that healthcare trainees receive comprehensive and up-to-date training. ICT plays a vital role in various aspects of medical education, spanning from content creation, presentation, dissemination, collaboration, and organization. A wide range of ICT tools have been employed in medical education, with ongoing evolution from ownership-based systems where educational materials are stored on diskettes, CDs, and hard disks to accessibility platforms through browsing or searchable online/offline materials. The Internet has been a catalyst in this evolution, leading to the implementation of learning management systems (such as Moodle, Blackboard, and Canvas) and the establishment of educational technology or media centres.

Although the traditional didactic lectures remain the primary method of instruction for knowledge transfer in most medical educational institutions including those in low-income countries [12], more newer instruction methods are available to supplement this. Methods such as the case-based, group-based student-led tutorials, and portfolio-based learning supplement didactic lectures in knowledge transfer. Moreover, clinical and procedural skills acquisition is facilitated through the traditional bedside teachings and supplemented by skill-based or case-based simulations.

All these learning methods can be enhanced through the integration of ICT inside the classroom and or clinics [13]. With the aid of audio-visual recordings, rare clinical cases or procedures can be archived and replayed multiple times offering learners invaluable learning opportunities. More advanced educational technologies can offer improved presentation features, including embedded videos, hyperlinks, and commands within presentations. They can also provide advanced tools such as audience engagement tools, writing screens, and screen capture methods, as well as enable collaborative annotation and leverage social media. For all these to be fully utilized in a low-income country such as Uganda, the ICT should be adaptable and accessible to both students and their instructors.

The theory of perceived attributes to innovation [14] can be used to illustrate the uptake of ICT innovation in medical education in LMICs. According to this theory, an individual is more likely to adopt a specific innovation if it possesses certain attributes. The theory proposed a five levels attribute that are illustrated in **Figure 1**.

2.3 Theory of perceived attribute to innovation

Comparative advantage refers to how much better an innovation is compared to existing technologies. Innovations that allow for reuse, redistribution, asynchronous access, and increased interactivity are more likely to be embraced by students and educators. Compatibility is key; technologies like lecture production gained popularity post-COVID-19 due to lecturers' familiarity with virtual platforms. The complexity of an innovation matters; simpler technologies like Zoom lectures are preferred over complex studio setups, impacting adoption rates. Triability, or the ease of trying out an innovation, plays a role in acceptance. Lastly, observable positive results increase the likelihood of adoption. In the realm of medical education, simplicity and familiarity are crucial for uptake of ICT platforms.

2.4 Electronic learning platforms

Electronic learning (e-learning) is one of the tools that has been embraced in these settings, its use intensified during the COVID 19 pandemic, and it covers a spectrum of activities involving use of technology to support parts of learning or instruct an entire curriculum [15]. In medical education, e-learning takes various approaches such as blended learning, Web-based learning, eTutor/eMentor programs, simulations, and use of multi-media software. These platforms leverage technology to tailor educational content based on the learner's progress, ensuring that the curriculum remains relevant and engaging. In resource-limited areas, where physical textbooks may be scarce, digital platforms offer a scalable solution, providing access to a vast array of medical resources.

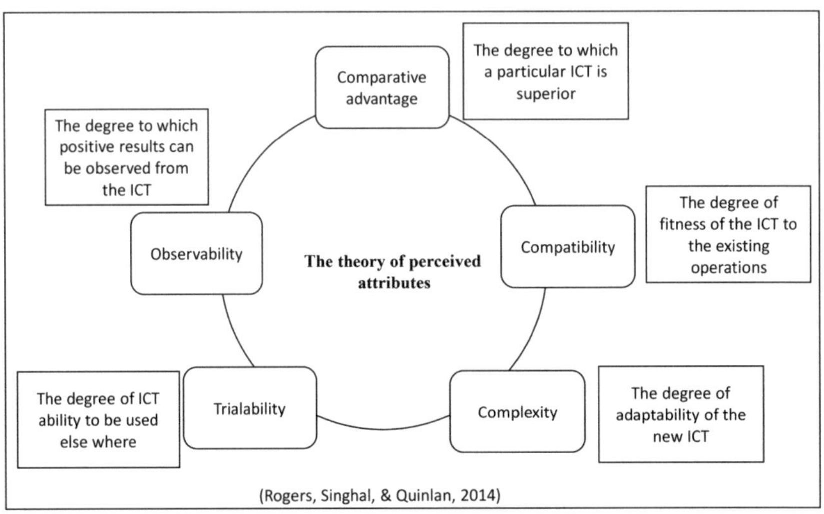

Figure 1.
Theory of perceive attribute to an innovation.

2.5 Mobile learning apps

Recognizing the widespread availability and affordability of smart mobile phones, the development of medical learning apps has proven to be one of the most effective means of instruction. Popular apps include Medscape, UpToDate, Coursera offers a flexible, convenient, and cost-effective learning platforms compared to paper-based approaches allowing students to access educational materials anytime and anywhere [8]. Additionally, interactive features such as quizzes, and virtual case studies enhance the learning experience, making complex medical concepts more digestible.

With increasing digitalization and technological enhancement in the learning Apps, medical educators and learners can benefit from both self-directed as well as collaborative learning. Literatures have shown that digital collaborative learning has better prospects in enhancing students' knowledge and competence compared to traditional methods of instruction. In a meta-analysis of five randomized control trials involving 647 nursing students, digital collaborative learning has been shown to enhance nursing students' interaction and collaborative skills, problem-solving skills, satisfaction, and motivation for learning [16]. Online or in-apps platforms that facilitate group discussions, collaborative projects, and knowledge sharing bridge the geographical gaps in resource-limited areas. These platforms also serve as a space for peer support and mentor, creating a sense of community among learners.

2.6 Artificial intelligence in medical education

In resource-limited settings, the integration of artificial intelligence (AI) into medical education is transformative, addressing enduring challenges and significantly improving the training of healthcare professionals [17]. AI technologies provide personalized and accessible learning experiences, with virtual simulations powered by AI algorithms offering crucial platforms for hands-on skills development. Overcoming resource constraints, these simulations facilitate repetitive practice, fostering mastery and confidence among medical students. The introduction of AI also introduces real-time feedback mechanisms, particularly valuable in settings where expert faculty is scarce. Embracing innovative technologies in resource-limited environments contributes to a more inclusive and equitable medical education landscape, and ensuring learners can access cutting-edge training resources regardless of geographical or financial constraints. As a seasoned medical and clinical educator, advocating for the strategic incorporation of AI into the curriculum becomes imperative for maintaining adaptive, effective, and globally accessible medical training [18].

Web-based and app-based AIs play an integral role in providing collaborative intelligence to enhance medical education [19]. These technologies seamlessly integrate with educational platforms, creating a collaborative ecosystem that enriches the overall educational journey for medical students. Augmented intelligence, facilitated by these AIs, assists learners in accessing extensive medical information, tailoring content to individual needs, and providing personalized study plans based on performance assessments. Within this collaborative intelligence framework, Web-based and app-based AIs foster interaction and engagement among learners, featuring interactive simulations, virtual case studies, and collaborative problem-solving exercises. By encouraging collaboration, these AIs simulate real-world medical scenarios, enabling students to work together, share insights, and collectively deepen their understanding of complex medical concepts. Consequently, Web-based and app-based AIs not only enhance individual intelligence but also cultivate collaborative intelligence, essential for teamwork and interdisciplinary communication in the medical field, optimizing the learning experience for future healthcare professionals [20].

2.7 Simulation-based technology

Simulation in medical education is a humane form of training in which learners are exposed to a controlled environment of real-life scenarios with room for learning from their mistakes. In resource-limited areas where resources for practical training may be scarce, simulations and virtual reality play key role. This not only supplements traditional training but also allows students to practice and refine their skills without the need for expensive equipment or cause harm to patients. The simulation environment encourages repetitive practice, constructive feedback, individualized learning, and variable clinical scenarios with defined outcomes [21].

Simulation may involve technology utilization and task complexity, aimed at equipping learners for clinical work, including managing workload and workflow [22]. It prepares students for the challenges they will encounter in real-world medical practice which include clinical skills, emergency response, communication skills, leadership initiatives and chain of command, critical thinking, problem-solving, decision-making, crisis response, and ethical considerations [23].

2.8 Simulation training at Gulu University in Uganda

Recognizing the crucial needs for the inclusion of technology into medical education, even in resource-limited settings [24] such as in Uganda, Gulu University Simulation Laboratory, was established in the Faculty of Medicine to offer a low-medium fidelity audio-visual simulations. More advanced technological option involved the use of a large interactive screen that links audio-visual simulation debriefs, the Web, and computer creating a seamless learning platform.

Gouzi et al. [25], illustrated the use of interactive screens as an essential tool for immersive medical training among undergraduate students. In their experiment, they engaged medical students in clinical reasoning exercises, where case scenarios, resulting clinical symptoms, tests, and hypotheses were mapped by students onto the interactive screen display. They found that learners demonstrated increased clinical reasoning [25]. This aligns seamlessly with simulation-based methodologies, emphasizing the critical need for such approaches in medical education. Our interactive screen **Figure 2** combines a display panel with touch-sensitive technology, enabling users to engage with digital content in a dynamic and hands-on manner. The device is versatile and surpasses traditional screens, projectors, or smart whiteboards, providing enhanced functionality and promoting engaging and collaborative user experiences. Its integration into the simulation technology has enabled us to provide a real-time audio-visual experience for both simulation and debrief sessions. This not only enhances trainees engagement but also transforms passive observation into active learning, fostering critical thinking, problem-solving, and skills acquisition.

The use of semi-automated medium fidelity manikins and high-quality recordings contribute to an immersive and effective participatory learning atmosphere. Post-simulation, the students that participated take centre stage during debriefing sessions, and their recorded sessions are played by the simulation assistant for critiquing. Thereafter, the team in the simulation room has the opportunity to share their experiences, lessons learned, and challenges they experienced—thereafter the faculty

DOI: http://dx.doi.org/10.5772/intechopen.115049

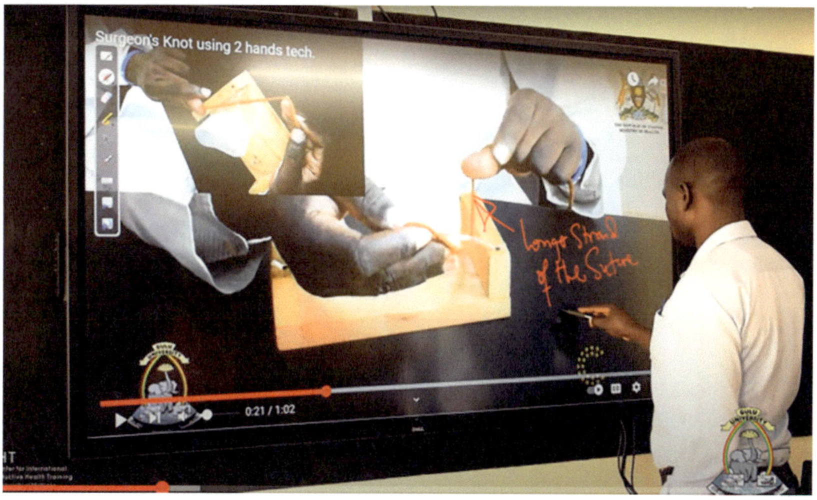

Figure 2.
Interactive screen being used during a simulation training to illustrate the process of knot tying.

together with the simulation assistants aid students to learn from their experiences, weakness and build on their clinical skills.

The interactive screen (**Figure 2**) emerges as powerful tool providing a platform for clear drawings and annotations and illustrations of information or procedures that are difficult to illustrate using the traditional display technology. This not only reforms medical education but also opens avenues for future research in medical education within resource constrained settings for innovative teaching methodologies. The intuitive touch interface simplifies navigation and interaction, making it user-friendly and accessible to individuals with varying technical proficiency just like a screen touch laptop and associated with better knowledge and skills retention due to active engagement as was described by Ref. [26].

2.9 Low-cost content production studio

Castillo and others in 2021 describe the process of how low-cost educational content is produced; the three phases are preproduction, production, and postproduction [27]. Although a variety of content recording options has been used ranging from simple setups, such as using a webcam and microphone, to more sophisticated setups with professional recording equipment and studios. Our experience in the production of content involved simple interface as illustrated in **Figures 3** and **4** below. The studio is configured to enable users capture video and audio signals using different sources of equipment enabling recording, livestreaming, storage, and playback of audio-visual signals (**Figure 3**). The production of content in the studio can vary depending on the context, platform, and the preferences of the faculty or instructor.

2.10 Content production setup

Our setup involves a simple but user-friendly recording design which integrates audio and video inputs to create a unique output. The video signals come from up to three different cameras depending on the complexity of the recording and the desires

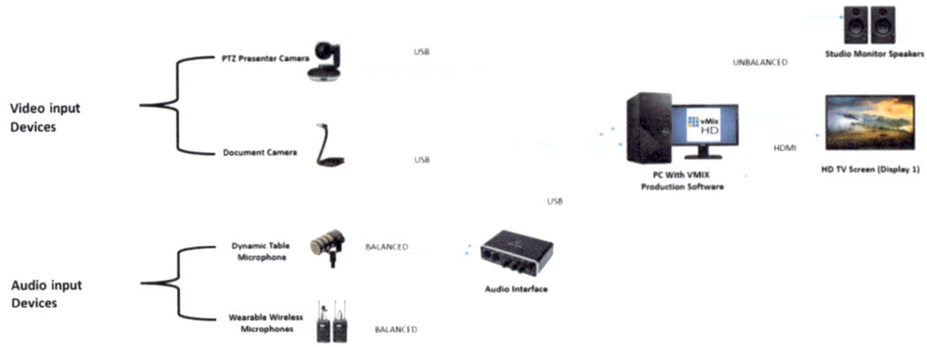

Figure 3.
Recording solution illustration.

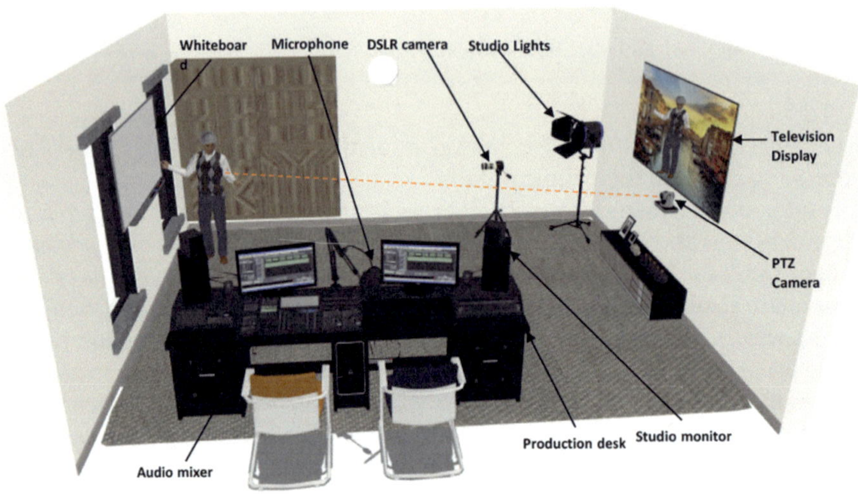

DSLR- Digital single lens reflex camera

Figure 4.
Artistic impression of the content production studio.

of the faculty in illustrating a particular detail. As illustrated in **Figure 3**, the video signals come from 1) document camera that captures video signals of different physical media like paper articles or illustration and objects and send them to the computer. 2) Pan Tilt and Zoom (PTZ)) camera, a dynamic tool controlled using a remote and can be used to pick video signals when a faculty is demonstrating or illustrating on whiteboards giving a feel of classroom setup. 3) Digital Single Lens Reflex (DSLR) camera is movable gadget that is varied depending on the direction of the video signals intended and can be used to record off studio contents.

The audio input sources comprise of dynamic unidirectional microphone for PowerPoints voiceovers and wireless microphone which can be worn by the user especially when they are making a presentation on the white board. All the microphone signals fed into the audio interface (**Figure 3**) before being relayed a computer for processing. The video and audio signals are integrated into a computer using a commercial Vmix production software. For controlled production, the audio-visual signals being recorded are relayed on to the television screen and sounds are monitored through studio monitors (**Figure 3**).

2.11 Content production process

Pre-production: Faculties typically start by outlining the topics they want to cover in their contents. They may write scripts, create slides, notes, or other materials to guide their presentation.

Production: Faculties may record their contents in a single take or break them down into smaller segments. With the help of additional mobile camera and a dedicated production assistant, clinical cases and procedures can be recorded even in wards or procedure rooms.

Postproduction: Post-production editing may be done to improve the overall quality of the contents. This involve removing redundant recordings, enhancing audio, or adding visual effects. Commercial editing software like Adobe Premiere, Movavi, or other video editing tools has been used as was elsewhere [28]. The editing is done either in the presence or under the guidance of the faculty involved in the production of the subject contents. The produced and edited contents are then uploaded to the chosen platform. This can be a learning management system (LMS), video hosting service like YouTube, or a specialized educational platform. In our case, the contents are uploaded in these two YouTube channels: https://youtube.com/@gusrhrcavstudio?si=85PZPB1-d2G6gV4x_and_UCumF7dQk1usZtzjZnHNOnhQ.

With online distribution platforms, educational contents produced in our studio is accessible to a global audience. This expands the reach of educational resources, reaching learners who may be geographically distant from traditional educational institutions. These innovative approaches can enhance the learning experience and provide students with a broader range of resources. Pre-recorded content saves time for educators who might otherwise spend a significant portion of class time on repetitive explanations. Additionally, it can be a cost-effective way to deliver high-quality learn ing materials without the need for continuous live presentations. Conclusively, the content production studio has the potential to positively impact learning by creating engaging, flexible, and inclusive educational content that aligns with diverse learning styles and preferences in low-income countries. This innovation is cost effective and user friendly and can be replicated in educational institutions in many settings.

3. Conclusion

The integration of ICTs in medical education offers a promising avenue to enhance learning experiences, promote student-centred approaches, and bridge educational gaps in healthcare training. The utilization of ICT tools like interactive displays, content production studios, and virtual simulations not only revolutionize content delivery but also foster critical thinking and problem-solving skills among students. While challenges such as the digital divide persist, efforts to leverage ICTs in medical education, as demonstrated in Ugandan contexts, exemplify the potential for technology to improve training outcomes and prepare healthcare professionals to meet the demands of a rapidly evolving healthcare landscape. Embracing innovative technologies and adapting teaching methodologies to accommodate diverse learning styles are crucial steps towards ensuring the competency and readiness of future healthcare providers.

Acknowledgements

Although this manuscript had no funding, the establishment of the simulation Laboratory and Lecture Production studio was supported with funding from the Center for International Reproductive Health Training at the University of Michigan (CIRHT-UM). The funder had no role in writing the manuscript.

Conflict of interest

The authors declare no conflict of interest.

Author details

Pebalo Francis Pebolo*, Ayikoru Jackline, Maxwell Opwonya, Raymond Otim and Felix Bongomin
Faculty of Medicine, Gulu University, Uganda

*Address all correspondence to: pebalopebolo@gmail.com

References

[1] Nicolaou C, Matsiola M, Kalliris G. Technology-enhanced learning and teaching methodologies through Audiovisual media. Education Sciences. 2019;**9**(3):196. DOI: 10.3390/educsci9030196

[2] Chase TJG et al. Mobile learning in medicine: An evaluation of attitudes and behaviours of medical students. BMC Medical Education. 2018;**18**(1):152

[3] Krathwohl DR. A revision of Bloom's taxonomy: An overview. Theory Into Practice. 2002;**41**(4):212-218

[4] Whillier S, Lystad RP. Intensive mode delivery of a neuroanatomy unit: Lower final grades but higher student satisfaction. Anatomical Sciences Education. 2013;**6**(5):286-293

[5] Dent JA. A Practical Guide for Medical Teachers. London, UK: Elsevier; 2017

[6] Jensen E. Teaching with the Brain in Mind. Alexandria, Virginia, USA: ASCD; 2005

[7] O'Doherty D et al. Barriers and solutions to online learning in medical education–an integrative review. BMC Medical Education. 2018;**18**(1):1-11

[8] Frehywot S et al. E-learning in medical education in resource constrained low-and middle-income countries. Human Resources for Health. 2013;**11**:1-15

[9] Rajab MH et al. Challenges to online medical education during the COVID-19 pandemic. Cureus. 2020;**12**(7)

[10] Lancaster LC, Stillman D. When generations collide: Who they are, why they clash, how to solve the generational puzzle at work. New York, USA: Harper Collins Business and economics; 2003. pp. 337-338

[11] Dolot A. The characteristics of generation Z. E-mentor. 2018;**74**(2):44-50

[12] Niccum BA et al. Innovation and entrepreneurship programs in US medical education: A landscape review and thematic analysis. Medical Education Online. 2017;**22**(1):1360722

[13] Cheng L, Ritzhaupt AD, Antonenko P. Effects of the flipped classroom instructional strategy on students' learning outcomes: A meta-analysis. Educational Technology Research and Development. 2019;**67**(4):793-824

[14] Rogers EM, Singhal A, Quinlan MM. Diffusion of innovations. In: An Integrated Approach to Communication Theory and Research. New York, USA: Routledge; 2014. pp. 432-448

[15] Lewis KO et al. Leveraging e-learning in medical education. Current Problems in Pediatric and Adolescent Health Care. 2014;**44**(6):150-163

[16] Männistö M et al. Digital collaborative learning in nursing education: A systematic review. Scandinavian Journal of Caring Sciences. 2020;**34**(2):280-292

[17] Wartman SA, Combs CD. Medical education must move from the information age to the age of artificial intelligence. Academic Medicine. 2018;**93**(8):1107-1109

[18] Mir MM et al. Application of artificial intelligence in medical

education: Current scenario and future perspectives. Journal of Advances in Medical Education & Professionalism. 2023;**11**(3):133

[19] Wang W. Medical education in China: Progress in the past 70 years and a vision for the future. BMC Medical Education. 2021;**21**(1):1-6

[20] Davenport T, Kalakota R. The potential for artificial intelligence in healthcare. Future Healthcare Journal. 2019;**6**(2):94

[21] Scalese RJ, Obeso VT, Issenberg SB. Simulation technology for skills training and competency assessment in medical education. Journal of General Internal Medicine. 2008;**23**:46-49

[22] Elshama SS. How to apply simulation-based learning in medical education? Iberoamerican Journal of Medicine. 2020;**2**(2):79-86

[23] Heidari M, Shahbazi S. Effect of training problem-solving skill on decision-making and critical thinking of personnel at medical emergencies. International Journal of Critical Illness and Injury Science. 2016;**6**(4):182

[24] Alenezi M, Wardat S, Akour M. The need of integrating digital education in higher education: Challenges and opportunities. Sustainability. 2023;**15**(6):4782

[25] Gouzi F et al. Interactive whiteboard use in clinical reasoning sessions to teach diagnostic test ordering and interpretation to undergraduate medical students. BMC Medical Education. 2019;**19**:1-13

[26] von Zadow U et al. SimMed: Combining simulation and interactive tabletops for medical education. In: Proceedings of the SIGCHI Conference on Human Factors in Computing Systems. New York, NY, United States: Association for Computing Machinery; 2013

[27] Castillo S et al. Production processes for creating educational videos. CBE—Life Sciences Education. 2021;**20**(2):es7

[28] Tejedor LC, Méndez JAJ, Palomera PR. Development of audiovisual material for teaching in medicine. In: Proceedings of the Second International Conference on Technological Ecosystems for Enhancing Multiculturality. New York, NY, United States: Association for Computing Machinery; 2014